Be Your Own Healer

Be Your Own Healer

*An Intuitive Doctor's Guide to
Activating Your Innate Abilities
Through MindBody Medicine*

Kim D'Eramo, DO

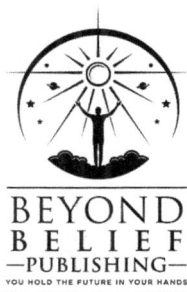

BEYOND
BELIEF
—PUBLISHING—
YOU HOLD THE FUTURE IN YOUR HANDS

ISBN: 978-1-957972-69-5

Dedicated to all the deeply empathic and heart-centered people who have come to assist humanity in awakening and who have suffered being here without a clue as to what is going on. I am grateful you are here with me. Now let's consciously create and have this all be so much more fun!

To all my past patients who have allowed me to learn through your journey. I could never have come through mine successfully without you.

PRAISE FOR
Be Your Own Healer

"*Be Your Own Healer* shows you how to scratch beneath the surface of your health in simple and easy ways that anyone can implement. Whether you have a mystery illness, an auto-immune illness, anxiety, or emotional distress, Dr. Kim D'Eramo will show you how to activate your healing power within!"

— Dondi Dahlin
International Bestselling Author of *The Five Elements*

"Thank you, Dr. D'Eramo, for a personal healing system that is both fascinating and action-oriented. This is a blessing for anyone wanting to experience healing for themselves and a 'must-read' for anyone looking to activate healing and personal power."

— Iyanla Vanzant
Multiple #1 NY Times Bestselling Author
Host of #1 reality show *Iyanla, Fix My Life* on Oprah
Winfrey Network (OWN)

"*Be Your Own Healer* is not merely a book; it's a beacon for anyone on a quest to activate their inner healing powers and harness their personal strength. Dr. D'Eramo masterfully guides readers through the complexities of the human body and mind, providing a clear path to wellness and empowerment. A seminal work for those ready to take control of their health journey."

— Nick Ortner
NY Times Bestselling Author of *The Tapping Solution*

"Dr. Kim D'Eramo shares her struggles, her triumphs and her transformation in a beautifully written insightful new book that gives all of us a fresh chance at personal empowerment."

— **Carol Look,** LCSW, DCH, EFT
Master and Author of *Attracting Abundance with EFT*

"**Be Your Own Healer** is a personal healing system that is a 'must-read' for anyone wanting to experience healing for themselves, or strengthen their ability to heal others. It is a roadmap to master healing for autoimmune illness, pain, anxiety or mystery illness, and should be mandatory reading for students and professionals alike!"

— **Dr. Peta Stapleton**
World Leading Clinical Psychologist, Educator
Author of *The Science Behind Tapping*

"Dr. Kim's inspiration to activate the healer within is contagious in **Be Your Own Healer**. Auto-immune illnesses, pain patterns, anxiety and more are addressed in a relatable, concise, and a straight-to-the-truth manner. Our humanity needs to lean in and educate themselves to the power within to heal. Here is a great place to do so! Thank you, Dr. Kim!"

— **Dr. Sue Morter**
Author of the Bestseller,
The Energy Codes: The Seven Step System to Awaken Your Spirit, Heal Your Body and Live Your Best Life
Founder of Morter Institute for Bio-Energetics,
LiveAwake!™ Year Long Study Program for Awakening
Founder of BodyAwake® School of Yoga
Co-Founder of Bio-Energetic Synchronization Technique
Host of Gaia TV's *Healing Matrix*

Contents

Acknowledgments   11
Foreword   13
Introduction   17
Activate Your Inner Healer   35

CHAPTER ONE
Tapping Into Infinite Power   37

CHAPTER TWO
You Are a Creator   67

CHAPTER THREE
Don't Believe What You Think   111

CHAPTER FOUR
Your Truth Is Written on Your Heart   157

CHAPTER FIVE
Let Your Biggest Problem Be Your Greatest Gift 193

CHAPTER SIX
Shift Your Consciousness to Shift Your Health –
Your 3-Step Process for Instant Healing   229

Conclusion   293
Next Steps   297
Let's Go Deeper   299
References   301
About the Author   303

Acknowledgments

Thank you to all of those who have made this book possible:

My mother for making me stronger;

My sister Kristen for always being my biggest cheerleader;

Laura Allahverdi, my manager, for partnering with me, being such a rock star, and always giving 200%;

My amazing business team for your devotion and excellence in the work we do;

All of my clients in Embracing Health and Be the Medicine, and everyone in the MindBody Community for being willing to be seen and to receive;

Ellen Rainford, who, as a receiver and a contributor, has made this a better book;

Jeri Ludwig, for being a nurturing presence of love in our home so we are free to be great parents and creators;

My sweet children, and my husband and soulmate, Mario, for being my foundation of so much love and power and my inspiration to let life be more awesome every day.

Foreword

I've been a proponent for conscious health for many years. Some of you may know me as an E! News host, others may have seen me introducing movies on theater screens or giving life tips on TVs at America's gas pumps. Maybe you've seen my work in the WWE, on the show *Bar Rescue*, or even in a Lifetime Christmas movie. Or maybe you know me for my health issues....

I'm no stranger to navigating and overcoming multiple health crises. It began nearly a decade ago, when my beloved mother was diagnosed with a stage 4 glioblastoma brain tumor. Months later in the ultimate irony, I was diagnosed with a brain tumor of my own—a meningioma tumor. We both underwent brain surgeries and my new life calling began: to help mom and myself heal and help others do the same. Mom sadly graduated to heaven. She was given months to live after her initial diagnosis, however, through alternate healing modalities, she lived five wonderful years.

My health journey was far from concluded as two years later, I was diagnosed with Type One Diabetes. In further irony, in the months following I discovered I had a stage 2 neuroendocrine tumor in my pancreas.

Today, I am here healthy and happy as a new mom, and completely cancer free. While western medicine has provided me with life changing surgeries and scans, I have relied on such things as increased sunlight, following circadian rhythms, limiting blue light, eating cleaner AND working on my mental health while applying meditation practices.

Since my brain tumor, I have dedicated my life and mission to getting better—and helping others to do the same. I altered my daily YouTube show and podcast from celebrity interviews to life and health improvement. On my Heal Squad series, I interview the greatest healers in order to explore and learn about new methods of healing. Though I'm not a doctor, since my brain tumor I have volunteer coached hundreds of others with tumors and cancer, proudly calling them my 'patients.' My one conclusion is that today more than ever we all must be the CEOs of our own health. The responsibility of healing rests upon us—and yes, we have the power to do so as ***Be Your Own Healer*** will show you!

Around the time of my diabetes diagnosis, I was introduced to Dr. Kim D'Eramo and her MindBody TV YouTube series. I had been working with Dr. Joe Dispenza, embracing the notion that if our minds can make us sick (they can) then why, logically, can't our minds heal us? (They can!) My husband, Keven, had become a weekly fan of Dr. Kim's series. Kev mentioned Dr. Kim shared in Dr. Joe's sentiments and that we should have her on the show. That's when I received the gift of meeting Dr. Kim.

Dr. Kim's assessment of my situation was spot on. They say when it comes to medicine and healing the motto is 'east meets west is best,' and with Dr. Kim, that's who you get. In addition to her mind body approach and osteopathic medical training, she was trained at Emory University, one of the top medical facilities in the United States and a Level I Trauma Center, and had years of experience as an emergency room physician. She literally IS east meets west! Dr. Kim's work is powerful. She also has a genuine, warm, loving, patient, empathetic and gentle bedside manner in her approach which helps even more.

My brain surgeon and friend, Dr. Keith Black, one of the smartest people I have ever met, shares that when it comes to the power of the mind to heal the body, we are just scratching the surface of what it can achieve. Dr. Kim's book not only brings you this depth of MindBody science, it also gives you practical tools and applications to be the CEO of your own health and help you and/or loved ones heal yourselves—which IS the future of healing and health care. Most doctors have but 20 minutes or less with you. That's all their packed schedules provide. Their intentions are most certainly good but can that fraction of time really be enough? It isn't. In addition to utilizing doctors, we must all take control of our own healing—including using our minds to help heal our bodies. That practice begins with adding this book to your library and then using it as a reference. We will all face health crises in our lifetimes, whether our own or a loved one's. Dr. Kim gives you the opportunity to navigate those situations with strength, power and certainty. May you use *Be Your Own Healer* and the information within it to get well. Here's to good health and good minds and bodies!

~Maria Menounos
New York Times Bestselling Author
American Television Reporter
Television Personality
Host of Heal Squad

Introduction

Can you really be your own healer?

You have a power inside you available to do unthinkable things. In this book I share the true nature of reality, in which, rather than being part of a solid, static, physical world, we exist in a matrix of pure energy. Everything you see is alive and conscious. All of what appears to be solid is in constant motion and flux—and it's impacted by you. Your consciousness has an impact on the world around you. In science, this is called the *observer effect*, and it's far more significant than most realize.

This means everything can change. Matter is pure energy, and it's responding to you. It can shift instantly depending on how you observe it. Your body is pure energy and it's listening to your thoughts. What you are thinking and who you are being are reflected in your body right now. This means to change what's going on in your body at the deepest levels, you must change your consciousness. This can happen instantly when you integrate the principles I share in this book.

For you to *be your own healer* and activate your innate power for healing, it is essential you are receptive to the following:

> Realize you *do* have the power within you to allow massive change.

> Adopt some new *innerstandings* you may have never considered before.

Let go of ideas you may have believed you needed to hold on to.

These will all be aligned with the highest Truth of nature and awaken you to something that's been within you all along.

This book is about new possibilities in medicine you may not have imagined that open you to potentials and powers within yourself. It's about creating a world where we all live in alignment with that truth and power.

We are releasing the old way of living, in which we believed our power and our value was outside ourselves and we looked to authorities for answers. We are coming into connection and communion within, where infinite wisdom lies. We are beginning to live according to that truth, and to create from the *inside out*. This allows us to craft previously unthinkable, extraordinary creations instead of operating from the template of what we think is true and what has already been established.

This book is an invitation to tap into that infinite source of healing, creation, and guidance within you to live a life of purpose, fulfillment, and contribution. This is the life you are meant to live. Within you lies the key to unlocking the resources for its creation.

I share with you new perspectives that open you to the deeper truth of reality and allow you to harness the power within you— the power from which you were created. This allows major and significant changes in your life. I also share a 3-step process I've been shown through accessing higher consciousness. I have used it throughout my life to witness the resolution of disease in myself and in others and to allow miracles that would have been thought to be impossible. Additionally, I've included links to several powerful audios, videos, and other materials to assist you in integrating this work.

Go to DrKimD.com/BYOHbonuses to access these powerful bonuses now!

If you've ever picked up on other people's energy, tuned into their emotions, or had awareness of what was going on in their systems, you know what it is like to be highly sensitive. Some people call this being *empathic*. I wasn't aware of that word until more recently, but I have been a deeply intuitive, empathic person throughout my life. For many years, I thought there was something wrong with me because others weren't aware of what I was perceiving. Very few people around me were awake to what was going on within themselves, but I could see easily. I thought others were lying when they pretended to be okay or pretended to be something they were not, but in fact, they simply weren't aware.

I realized after a time, most other people were so disconnected from their inner world and their emotions, thoughts, and beliefs that they were robotically living out a program of who they had learned they were supposed to be. They were following the blueprint of the program and not living in accordance with their True-Selves. I realized my ability to sense what was happening in myself and others—to hear thoughts and feel emotions—did not need to be a problem and did not mean something was wrong with me. I realized it could be an asset—a superpower—if I could let it serve a higher purpose. I also realized this was not something that was meant to serve only *me*. I was created with these abilities because I was meant to share this profound awareness as a gift.

In my teens, I had a powerful awakening experience during which my intuitive gifts were greatly amplified. I could see what was going to happen just before it happened, could hear people's thoughts, and could know what they were about to say before they spoke. I could witness how my thoughts and beliefs immediately impacted the physical energies and people around me. I saw my own thoughts and ideas instantly reflected in what others said or did or in the sounds and events taking place around me. I felt and sensed a profound connection with everyone and everything. During this experience, the barriers of separation dissolved.

I felt scared of this; I did not understand what was happening. For years I experienced intermittent bouts of panic because it was such a major change in my whole foundation of reality. I had previously seen myself as a solid, separate self and believed I could only know things through direct experience. This experience in Oneness consciousness wasn't anything I had ever learned about, but it was far more real than anything I'd ever experienced in the illusory world of separation I had been living in until that time. I recognized that I was connected with everyone and everything and could know things beyond the solid and separate self I had thought myself to be.

That experience took years to fully integrate. I grew up in the Boston area in a Catholic family who basically left the spiritual stuff up to the priest and believed everything the doctor said; I'd learned not to question reality. It took me a long time to integrate my spiritual experience, trust my inner knowing, and let this heightened awareness become a gift and not a curse.

At that time, I knew I was here to share profound truths with the world—we are creative, we have the power to manifest reality, and we are each intimately connected with the world around us and with the Divinity within ourselves.

I developed an understanding that the way the world viewed disease was a very, very limited way of seeing what was happening. We were looking at the tip of the iceberg—the physical symptoms—rather than the underlying energy that manifests disease.

I could see what was going on beneath the surface to create someone's disease, symptoms, problems, and challenges. I was shown a vision of how my life would play out. I would become a physician educated in Western medicine, and from that platform, I would share this truth in a meaningful way that would change the face of medicine. I had no idea how this would take place, but I was completely certain that the path would be laid out for me, and I was completely devoted to following it.

I later learned about osteopathic medicine and knew this would be part of my educational journey. In osteopathy, we learn about general medicine, surgery, pathology, and disease; we also learn about how the body heals itself and how the mind and body are connected. Through osteopathic training, I worked with amazing physicians who were doing incredible things I had not known were possible. They had the ability to sense and feel things from across the room, to guide and instruct people without touching their body, to know what had happened in someone's past without having met that person before. They could indirectly let in awareness and guide healing.

After seeing so many examples of this and witnessing so many people heal, I was deeply moved to operate this way as a physician and to go beyond seeing my patient as only a physical, separate being. I learned how to let in information and Intelligence that would serve the healing process, and to let that healing power guide me as I worked with my patients.

With all this understanding, plus the years of study I had already done in MindBody Medicine, one would think I was invincible to any illness that might come my way. Not so. During my second year of medical school, I began developing strange symptoms. I had severe joint pain, fatigue and lethargy, migraine headaches, and intermittent chills and body aches. I visited many doctors over the course of a year, and no one had an answer or solution. I struggled to overcome this illness and not let it get me down. I tried ignoring the fatigue and pushing through. I tried running through my severe joint pain.

Knowing that my body responds to my thoughts, I, of course, tried *mind-over-matter* approaches, to no avail. *The more I tried to heal, the worse and more complex my illness became.* During this time, I had to let go of everything I thought I understood about self-healing. I could not heal myself; I could only let go and allow the circumstances to take place that would allow my body to heal. This took a level of surrender I could not have learned from a book, and it changed the course of my life. The healing that happened, which I share in this book, strengthened the foundation of who I was here to be as a leader and physician.

During medical school, I applied for and was granted an osteopathic fellowship position, an extra year of medical training to learn osteopathy more fully and to study with amazing healers. I later went on to do my residency training in trauma and critical care as an emergency physician. I chose to do my residency training in Emergency Medicine because it was the only thing I could imagine doing in the conventional medical system. This may seem like the polar opposite of MindBody Medicine and osteopathic healing work, but my training as an Emergency Medicine doctor greatly served the healing work that I am doing now. Working in the emergency room required me to find a strong center of certainty and inner connection, so I could operate in clarity under the most intense and extreme life-and-death situations.

I learned that clamping down into fight-or-flight mode was the last thing that was going to help me in my work as an ER doctor. Rather, bringing more fluid breath to my body and connecting with my body would allow me to have greater power—whether it was seamless communication with my team, effortless calculations of medication doses, or full awareness of the time interval that had passed before needing to give the next dose of a drug during a resuscitation. I found when I slowed down my nervous system and connected within, I always had exactly what I needed, exactly when I needed it. Through this training, I entered into a deeper level of trust in my own intelligence.

My experiences in the ER inspired me to create the practice of medicine I am doing now. When someone would come in with a chronic ailment, I was able to sense the source of their illness, their pain, or their chronic symptoms. I knew if they understood what I was seeing, they could alleviate their illness without medications and without needing to return again and again to the Emergency Room. I felt deeply inspired to teach people about how their thoughts and emotions were keeping illness in place and how they could shift things by releasing the way they saw themselves and their symptoms. I would sometimes share my insights, and patients would be deeply grateful—sometimes moved to tears—because something within them knew what I was saying was true.

One woman named Eliza came to the ER with severe abdominal pain and a history of Crohn's disease—an inflammatory bowel disease known to be triggered by foods, by stress, and by unknown causes. I was given a notice by my staff that she was "drug seeking," which indicated she'd come for pain medication and was familiar to the team for similar past ER visits. Eliza had a desperate expression as she shared her story of how long this had been going on and that in the past few days she *just couldn't take it anymore* and *had to come in.* I could feel her distress and was curious to see whether there were underlying emotions we could release that would assist her healing. I probed into her relationships and home life.

"Are there any things going on at home that could have stressed you out and triggered this inflammation?" I asked.

She began tearing up. "I'm overwhelmed." She said. "No one understands how I feel. I have to take care of everything, and they think I'm crazy for having so much pain. I'm trying to tell them this is real and I can't do anything about it."

Whenever someone is arguing for their victimhood, it's a sure sign there is a deeper need asking to be met and there hasn't been an effective way to do it. They've bought into their own powerlessness and usually the hopelessness of their situation and are trying to get their needs met through that filter. It won't work when we do this. We'll just keep being more of a victim, more in lack, more in illness or poverty, but since we're typically not aware we're doing this, we just keep trying harder to make it work.

I asked her, "What if you didn't have to take care of everyone else?" She seemed a little taken aback.

She finally said, "I would have no purpose. I wouldn't know who I am. I don't have a career, and my husband takes care of me, so I have to give back. I have to have a role."

Now we were unwinding the core of what was going on. Eliza saw herself as a burden and needed to prove her worth by taking care of others, putting their needs first and ignoring her own. The illness was a way for her needs for self-care to surface and, on some level, to be met. Unconsciously, her need to let love in and be taken care of finally trumped the need to hold things together for everyone else.

The unconscious always prioritizes our greatest needs. Even though we may consciously want to get out of pain or illness, keep the family happy, or make money, the unconscious will let all of that go to meet the true priority: opening the system back up to love and Life Force.

I asked her, "How might this situation be serving you? If it did have a purpose, how might being sick be getting some of your needs met?"

This can be a difficult thing to consider, especially when someone is in so much pain or terror from their disease or feels guilty for being a burden on others, but I knew she felt my compassion and was ready to look at this.

"Well, I get to take a break and let everyone else go. I get to try to have them see and acknowledge that I have needs too."

". . . but it's maybe not going about it the best way, is it?" I offered. "Are you willing to make some changes and have a conversation with your family, so you can get your needs met *on* the table, instead of having it be under the table?"

She cried and was clearly aware that what we were uncovering was true. She wasn't sure how this would all work out, but she had uncovered the pattern, and the rest would unwind from there.

It was moments like these when I so strongly wanted to carve out a medical practice where I could really do the deep healing work. In the ER, there was barely space for this. I had just a few minutes with her, and dropping into this level of sensitivity was very difficult in the environment I was operating in. Working fast, thinking fast, moving people through, and checking the boxes to get them treated was a different way of operating that shut down my sensitivity and insight. Turning it on and off was highly destabilizing.

Most people coming to the ER weren't interested in the deeper truth. They wanted to get a quick fix and get back to their regularly scheduled lives. They weren't ready to hear what I was seeing or to step into true healing. I knew I ultimately wanted to be in a structure that was more supportive of my doing the deeper work.

After a couple of years of practicing full-time emergency medicine, I was exhausted. Almost daily I was praying: *Please God, get me out of here! Show me the way! I'll do anything!*

Repeatedly, I heard: *Be anxious for nothing. It's all coming to you.*

And I'd have a feeling of lightness and certainty for a while. This lasted until the next time I became overwhelmed and started dreading my situation: *I'll knock on doors to find office space and create a healing practice. I'll do whatever I have to do to make this work*, I would desperately think. Over and over again it was the same message: *Be still and know. It's all taken care of.*

The answer finally came in the form of an invitation to teach at an osteopathic medical school that was opening in Tennessee. That is where my two worlds came together. I moved to a peaceful, rural, beautiful place in the middle of nowhere. After my hectic life in Atlanta, this new environment shifted my nervous system into a state of calm and peace where I could integrate my life from a whole new vantage point. A few years after being part of that community, teaching incredible students and working with amazing doctors, I was inspired to move back to Boston where I had grown up. I did some shifts in the ER and started my osteopathic practice. This is when I finally began a practice using empowerment and awakening as a way to invite health back into the body.

That was the foundation for the work I am doing now. After seeing thousands of patients, I realized they all had the same root causes for illness, injuries, and pain: They were disconnected from their bodies and were afraid of their body and their symptoms. The symptoms were seen as a problem to be fixed, not a message for inner modification on their part. They couldn't feel the wisdom within calling out for change. I saw one person after another experience massive changes in their lives when they began to embrace this new perspective that Life was on their side.

I had so much to share, but it was heavy trying to do this one patient at a time, so I developed courses and programs and began teaching groups of people. The course was called *Empowerment for Total Wellness*, and it contained all the insights I'd had about how we are pure energy, we are self-healing, and symptoms are the body communicating with us. People loved the courses and the word spread. I brought that work online and shared it with larger groups of people. I have found every year there are more and more people inspired by this approach and open to a new perspective. Many of these people have the kind of pathologies that Western medicine has no answers for, such as fibromyalgia, chronic fatigue syndrome, or Hashimoto's thyroiditis; persistent progressive illnesses, such as cancer, pain syndromes, or digestive problems; autoimmune diseases such as multiple sclerosis (MS), an often-debilitating autoimmune disease that affects the nervous system; or neuropathic diseases.

There is a sort of wastebasket for these cases under the umbrella sentiment of: *We have a diagnosis for you but no clue as to why you have this problem or what to do about it.* Most doctors are overwhelmed handling cases such as these because they feel powerless to help. Patients with these conditions were my favorite to work with because I had a way to help them resolve their illnesses.

I understood exactly what was going on. I could read the body; I even had a sense of their history or their traumas or lineage patterns that were living in their systems, written on their DNA and creating these diseases. I could offer them simple ways to emerge beyond their diagnosis and create a new pattern of health.

I began passionately teaching these skills, and by the grace of God, my practice has grown internationally. Now, people all over the world interested in exploring new possibilities for healing can learn:

> We are not physically separate selves, but we are, in fact, energy.

> Our consciousness affects our bodies.

> Subtle shifts in our beliefs and emotions can create massive and profound shifts in our physical bodies and health.

> We can assist the healing process for ourselves and others.

I am grateful to be sharing the understanding I have gained through my work with my patients and clients, my medical training, and my personal journey with illness. I will share with you how to come into greater connection with your power for resolving disease, dissolving major problems and challenges in your life and unlocking your life force so you live freely.

I wrote my first book, *The MindBody Toolkit*, to share everything I had studied about MindBody healing, how the body heals itself, and what incredible things can happen when we ignite inner alignment.

I was on my own to figure out what to do with all the information I had learned about MindBody healing. We had the science and the studies; we understood the mind and body were connected and the body could heal itself, but I wanted to know: *What do I do to ignite those factors? What do I do to create those circumstances that allow spontaneous resolution of disease?*

In *The MindBody Toolkit*, I share ten tools that will help you instantly increase your energy, enhance productivity, and even reverse disease. I share ways to shift your frequency and shift your consciousness for the purpose of shifting your health. This second book is an extension of those skills. In this book, we go deeper into an understanding that your consciousness, your beliefs, and your emotions not only affect your body, your cells, and your DNA, but they also *extend beyond your body* and affect everything you create in your life. You are a creator.

Your consciousness, beliefs, and emotions affect:

Other people

Your circumstances

Whether opportunities arise in your life or elude you

Whether doors open before your eyes or they stay closed and you have to struggle

How you feel in each moment

How others perceive you and treat you

Every aspect of your life circumstances

In this book, you learn how to ignite the power within you for physical shifts and changes and to change the material conditions of your life. You are meant to live in peace, prosperity, love, and connection and to share your deepest gifts as a contribution to others. Together, when we embrace and embody this, we can create heaven on Earth.

This book is written for you who are ready to awaken beyond the paradigm of what you think is true, what you have been told, what you have learned—the way everybody else does it. This book is for you who know something else is possible, even though it may not appear in your life right now. *If you are ready to experience your true power and let in something way beyond what most people think is possible, this book is for you.*

Are you beginning to awaken to a deeper aspect of self through a chronic illness, a life-threatening situation, or a life-changing experience?

Are you awakening to the possibility of a life beyond lack, limitation, and sickness—beyond the ideas that life is a struggle and you always have to work hard?

Are you ready to let in something higher?

More and more of us are becoming sensitive and empathic, picking up on other people's emotions or energy. Because we experience conditions and sensations intensely, this can feel wrong to us or like a disease. It can feel like a curse and a limitation. Sometimes, we have to be careful around—or completely avoid—certain people or places. If you feel you have to be protected to get through your day, I am here to share that your heightened sensitivity is meant to be a gift.

If you are ready to trust the source within you and your innate gifts and abilities, letting them be a blessing instead of a curse, I'm glad you are here. If you realize you are meant to be not just surviving and managing the situation you are in, but also expanding beyond that and inviting everyone around you to do the same, this book is for you.

As you read this book, instead of approaching the content as more stuff to learn or something to implement later on with the hope of getting future results, I invite you to relax and soften. Do not try to understand this as you read; just be willing to let it in. Let the words and concepts work on you. Read the whole book or certain passages again to let the message sink in even deeper. If you let the body soften, relax, and breathe as you read, the gifts and Intelligence within you will awaken.

I hope you gain the ability to recognize within yourself something that goes beyond your understanding or your ability to control. We don't often want to give up control; however, there is something beyond the small-self that will fuel us, resource us, and fulfill us when we finally let go and allow it.

The power within you that heals your body activates and opens new possibilities in your life and shows you the way to a new reality. Let this book open that space in you that *does* know, because the greatest book or teacher is not the one who teaches you more information; they are the ones who point you to a deeper connection with the Divinity and Infinite Truth that already lives within you.

Activate Your Inner Healer

I am devoted to assisting you in awakening to your highest creative potential and living in true vitality. I've created bonuses along with this book for those seeking healing and those providing true healing modalities so we create this reality together.

Access the support bonuses now:

DrKimD.com/BYOHbonuses

CHAPTER ONE

Tapping Into Infinite Power

THE REAL REASON PEOPLE STAY STUCK

Many of us are dealing with problems we do not know how to handle—a health condition that does not have a solution, or a relationship challenge that is a conundrum and repeats itself, or maybe a job or money problem where there seems to be no way out. We do not realize our thinking and our perception propagate those negative and difficult patterns in our lives. It is not the external thing or an external reality we have to fix, but something that is happening within us.

Most of us have a limited understanding of what we truly are. We think the body is a physical, solid thing and that a disease is happening *to* us. We do not realize that this perspective—seeing ourselves as separate and at the mercy of our outer situations—creates how our physiology functions and how our body manifests.

The combination of our thinking and our perception—our way of seeing the world—creates a pattern that determines everything happening in our body. Our thoughts trigger a myriad of chemical processes, neurological messages, and electromagnetic signals that profoundly affect all of our physiology and brain functions. Just like a computer program, these patterns play on automatic pilot in the background while we're busy tending to other things.

The program: *I always have to do more* can send constant stress and inflammatory signals to the body, gearing you up for hyperdrive, for example. It may seem that some programs can be helpful to keep us protected from danger we've previously encountered, such as: *I should never trust anyone.* This program may have been helpful at one point during our life, such as during childhood or a time we experienced something harmful or traumatic. However, this programming consumes massive amounts of energy and doesn't serve us in the situation we are in now.

Many of us have created faulty programming about our powerlessness or helplessness that ends up looking something like:

> *I am a victim of my disease.*
>
> *There is nothing that can be done for my diagnosis.*
>
> *I have to be on medication.*
>
> *I'll never get better.*
>
> *I'm tired because I have_____* (fill in the blank with symptom/diagnosis).
>
> *The older I get, the harder I have to work to be healthy.*
>
> *After a certain age, things start to fall apart.*

Or programs not directly related to our health, such as:

There's no one out there for me.

Money does not grow on trees.

I need to work hard to have wealth.

I must have a degree to make a good living.

I can't do what I really love because no one will pay me for it.

I need to uphold my obligations and not let others down.

These faulty programs can keep us from making choices that could bring us great joy and prosperity. They prompt us to make choices that keep us limited, like staying in a job we hate because deep down we believe it won't be okay if we leave.

These unconscious programs create physiologic changes that cause inflammation, cellular discord, genetic mutation, and ultimately disease. These beliefs not only affect us physically, but they also change our electromagnetic field. That's because the body is made of energy, not physical material. As energy, it emits an energy field that can be sensed several feet away from the physical body. This energy field has electrical and magnetic qualities, which is why it is called the *electromagnetic field*. I elaborate on this more later in this book. The electromagnetic field correlates with your thought processes and governs everything in your body and mind.

I do all my work using the principles of MindBody Medicine because I have come to see that the *metaphysical*, or "that which governs the physical," is a far greater leverage point with which to impact someone's health, body, and life.

You Are Pure Energy, Not a Solid

Some of the limited understandings we have developed are:

- The body is purely physical.

- An illness is a physical thing that happens to us.

- Illness is our natural state; we can't live in a world without disease.

There has been a deeper reality uncovered in the field of quantum physics, where we study the smallest fundamentals that make up our body and world.

We have seen that cells are made of molecules and molecules are made of atoms. We set up models to examine the molecular structures, and everything seems very orderly and predictable. This is the model for classical mechanics, or *Newtonian physics*, in which we live in a universe unaffected by our participation with it. Newtonian physics says the universe behaves in predictable ways we can count on that are reproducible, unchanging, and unaffected by our observation of them.

When we explore how atoms and parts of atoms actually behave, however, the classical model of physics breaks down. Our apparently physical reality is not solid at all. When we observe the smallest particles that make up the world, we see the Universe is a *conscious field of energy*, not physical matter held within empty space.

Through the field of quantum physics, we witness the smallest particles that make up matter are more empty space than physical material. What appears to be solid is actually more than 99.999% empty space. In fact, according to calculations by Professors Stephen Hawking and Neil Turok's Theory of Open Inflation, if all the matter in the expanding Universe were compressed, the actual physical *stuff* would fit into a space the size of *one green pea*.

Of course, we see it as stuff; we do not realize we are in an almost completely empty space, a vibrating field of energy. Nor do we realize that field is responding to our observation of it. Quantum physics demonstrates the very act of simply looking at something—focusing our awareness upon it for even a moment—changes the properties of what that matter is doing on a quantum level.

Experiments in quantum physics have shown that changes in the *electrical* field surrounding an atom change the structure and activity of that atom. In scientific terms, this is known as the *Stark effect*. Science has also demonstrated that if we change the *magnetic* field around an atom, this generates changes in the function and activity of that atom. This is called the *Zeeman effect*. As I share later, your heart is the strongest electromagnetic field in your body, governing the state of all the atoms, molecules, cells, and organs of your body. You have the capacity to shift that electromagnetic field in favor of healing.

The energy field that matter is within is the most powerful force determining its properties and behavior. Our consciousness literally generates an energy field. Our thoughts and emotions directly influence the foundation of material reality around us.

I studied quantum physics in college, and I was dumbfounded. *Do you know what this means?!* I would think. I couldn't understand how my professor could put his pants on the same way every day and just go about life as if this was no big deal. I was utterly blown away when I saw how science had fully demonstrated the fluid and ever-changing nature of our material reality and how everything was affected by our observation of it. Everything truly is possible.

> *If quantum physics doesn't utterly shock you,*
> *you haven't understood it yet.*
>
> ~ Neihls Bohr

The foundation of conventional medical science is faulty. The belief that material reality is a solid, static, separate phenomenon is not true. It is the Newtonian perspective that the Universe is made of solid things that move and act in predictable ways, uninfluenced by our thoughts and observation is false. We see definitively through the study of quantum particles that this is not the case.

The materials of the Universe are not solid, static, or separate, and they are directly and immediately impacted by our thoughts and observations of them. The *stuff* we see is almost completely space. It's like looking at the Milky Way from a great distance. It looks like a thing, a swirl, a shape from far away—but zoom in, and we see the particles that make up the Milky Way are infinitely far apart from each other. There is far more space than stuff, and the thing that looked like a structure has no actual substance.

This is also true on the quantum level. The wooden table that looks solid is made up of particles which, when greatly magnified, are seen to be infinitely far apart, so much so that these particles are just potentials, pure energy, always moving and changing and impacted by the energy and space around them. When we view the table at the quantum level, we see it is almost completely made up of empty space.

The same goes for our physical body. What seems to be physical is pure energy. It is constantly moving, constantly changing, constantly shifting, and it is responding to us. It is responding to our thoughts, feelings, and ideas about it. Many ancient fields of medicine have known this all along, and those in the mainstream consciousness are now beginning to catch on.

If you wish to understand the Universe,
think in terms of energy, frequency, and vibration.
~ Nicola Tesla

Albert Einstein, Nicola Tesla, Niels Bohr, Max Plank, J. Robert Oppenheimer, Schrödinger, and many other scientists have conclusively demonstrated that the predictable, systematic laws of Newtonian physics are not the absolute rule about how our reality really functions. We are not in a physical universe.

Are you ready to let that concept in and operate differently?

Does that idea scare you? Confuse you? Make you feel insignificant?

What, if anything, would you let hold you back from embracing this new perspective?

The natural laws of how the body works break down when we witness remote healing—in which a person facilitates healing on an individual who is not in the same physical space; in fact, the practitioner and the client could be thousands of miles apart—or when we think of someone, and a few minutes later they call. Just last week when I was working on this book, my husband asked me about one of our assistants overseas.

He said, "You should call Carla."

I explained I was already in regular communication with her online.

"No," he said, "you need to call her and have a conversation."

A week later, there we were in Zoom to chat, and she shared with me that she was in a major life crisis over her relationship. She had been so overwhelmed, she was unable to work as she usually did, and I was one of the two clients she had kept. I shared some insights, and she broke down crying.

"This is exactly what I needed to hear," she said. "I know this is true, and I know what I need to do."

Within a week, she made a major change in that relationship and was ready to pick up more clients again. She later told me our conversation changed the course of her life.

So how is it we can connect with someone on the other side of the world when our current paradigm says that's impossible? Hmm . . . could those ideas about our physical reality be wrong?

We are not separate, and we are not primarily physical. The apparent boundaries of our body are not real; they're illusory.

I've given myself full permission to operate beyond those apparent boundaries and to function in a more expansive way in how I think, how I see those I work with, and how I interact with my world. As a result, I've witnessed hundreds of remote healings with people I've worked with. It's become so common, it doesn't even surprise me.

I once felt moved to send a text to a client to encourage her: "Let go of fighting. You can soften into your body, and all really will be well."

She was blown away to receive that message at the exact moment she was about to walk into a courtroom to contest allegations from her ex-husband who was threatening to take custody of her daughter. She did her best to soften and breathe fully, to surrender and trust. She later informed me the judge had thrown the case out after receiving evidence of her ex's overt lies related to the case.

What Is **Intuition** and Can We All Tap Into It?

Intuitive functions can seem strange to those who think we only access information through our five senses. However, there are many documented examples of a person knowing the exact moment something happened that was remote; for example, a loved one dying or being in a significant accident. Such an event occurred to the mother of author Mona Lisa Shultz, a prominent medical intuitive. She stood up during a meeting in front of a room full of people and screamed that her daughter was in trouble. The time had been documented in the minutes of the meeting. Later they found out it was the precise moment Mona Lisa had been in a car accident.

She wrote about it in her book *Awakening Intuition* (Bantam, 1999), which I devoured during medical school.

Have you ever experienced something like this or had a thought of someone, and then they called you, or felt inspired to reach out to someone and they told you *I was just thinking about you?* This happens all the time for members of my family and me. Being tuned in intuitively is something we can develop when we allow ourselves to function this way.

None of this can be explained from the understanding that we live in a purely physical universe and we are nothing but separate physical bodies. However, when we understand we are pure energy—that we are Intelligence and we are connected—remote healing, nonlocal communication, and spontaneous resolution of disease make total sense. We can receive information we would not have known from direct learning. When we are willing to let in information that goes beyond what the five senses alone would allow us to see and experience, we can surpass our limited physical experience. We can have an effect on others that the physical dimension does not allow for.

Your Electromagnetic Field

It seems the body ends at the barrier of the skin. However, the energy body does not end there, and neither does its impact. The HeartMath Institute has done extensive research to measure the electromagnetic field of the body. They've demonstrated the body emits both electrical and magnetic signals that can be measured up to ten feet away from the physical body. The strongest electromagnetic center in the body is the *heart*. This energy center is the area where we merge thought and emotion and generate *feeling*. The heart center is where thought and emotion come together, and this generates power. We will work with this more later in this book.

When we consider the body's electromagnetic field extends out beyond the body, it's easy to understand how our intention can induce nonlocal effects. People feel you. This impact occurs whether we are aware of it or not, but it can become more conscious and intentional: you can cultivate your personal power such that you generate the impact you truly want on your body, your life, and your world.

The body's electromagnetic field has a particular vibration that correlates with a person's emotional state. When we are in lower emotional states, such as anger or hatred, the vibrational frequency is slower and denser. When we're in the higher emotional states of love or joy, the vibrational frequency is faster and lighter.

Our electromagnetic signal affects everything going on within our physical body and impacts even other bodies around us. A person's physiology can change measurably when the surrounding vibration is changed. The person may become consciously aware of it and sense a "negative" or a "positive" person, or they may subconsciously avoid or gravitate toward a person. Whether a person is aware of the vibrational frequency of the people around them or not, their body *is*, and it will respond.

Some people are energy-sensitive and will feel when someone is harboring strong negative emotions. Most children have this capability. Others may move away from a person holding negative emotions but not know why. Still others engage the same way with the person, dismissing their own inner signals that their interactions could be detrimental.

When we are in higher emotional states—such as love, joy, or peace—our health and our physiologic function benefit. That higher-frequency field impacts our cells in a positive way and positively impacts everything around us. People want to be with us, life goes more smoothly, and we tend to bring out the best in others. Others may consciously note this and say: *I feel good around you*, or: *I like you*, or they may act more jovial and not be aware of it. Whether a person is aware of it consciously or not, a person in a *positive* electromagnetic state has a direct impact on others' well-being, mood, and body.

The opposite is true of a lower-frequency electromagnetic field. When we are harboring anger, jealousy, frustration, or shame, this has a hindering effect on our health. Our field negatively impacts the world around us. Just as when we are around someone in a lower frequency, our body registers it.

This is not to say others are victims of your lower emotions, nor are you of theirs. It's how we respond to that lower-frequency field—what we do with the awareness—that determines the outcome. We can react, reject, protect against, or run away from our own or others' negativity, or we can soften into the awareness and embrace it, allowing the deeper wisdom to emerge and show us a new way of being. This is how we evolve. Since our observation of matter directly and instantaneously affects how that matter behaves, this is an opportunity to practice compassion, so we can have a healing impact.

No Separation

Matter is not separate or independent from us. We impact it and are impacted by it. When we understand we are energy impacting energy, we understand we can impact everyone and everything around us. We go beyond the finite reality we appear to be in and move into an infinite reality with multiple potentials. Everything is connected. Even when particles are separated by miles, they are somehow still connected and instantaneously communicating information. Einstein's term for this phenomenon has been translated roughly from German to "spooky action at a distance."

When we see we are pure energy, not a solid, finite object, we make space for many more possibilities of how our cells respond when something like disease emerges. Let's say someone has cancerous liver cells. Through a minor shift in their energy field, those cells can rearrange themselves into healthy, vibrant liver cells. That quantum shift between a diseased cell and a healthy cell is a subtle tweak we allow. When we remember we are pure energy, when we live this way, we no longer see everything as a threat we need to fight against or flee. We know we are affected by the thoughts and expectations we hold, and we are affected by the energy field around us, so we find ways to shift those unwanted circumstances.

Ancient cultures have understood the truth: We are interconnected, and this apparently physical world is, in fact, a reflection of the consciousness within us. Many aboriginal cultures tune into their inner listening for guidance and survival. Their ability to know where to find food, where to set up their communities, and when to move their villages to avoid attack is based on this capacity for deep listening. Animals do the same. They tune into the electromagnetic field and let it guide them. They know when and where to migrate. They move together as one. You can see the effects of the field when you watch a school of fish all turn to the same direction in one instant. You can see this when birds fly in unison. This field is all around us, and we, as humans, can also tune into our inner connection to support us in every aspect of our lives.

Our culture has been vastly disconnected from any inner connection and instead has looked to the external to point us to the truth. We lead lives of conditional well-being in which we feel we must achieve more, purchase more, and control more in an ineffective attempt to secure our well-being. Rather than see we are infinitely provided for and can tune within for guidance, we've largely given authority figures the power and looked to them to tell us what to do. We've come further and further from our connection within and our inner authority. This approach will always backfire as life continuously tries to lead us back to the true source of power.

If everything is governed by frequency and consciousness, and the material stuff is infinitesimally small compared to the space of the field it resides in, do you see how *stuff* can change significantly with a minor change in the frequency of the field?

This is how you can let your life change instantly. Depending on the frequency of the field, the *stuff* arises either as a life-giving, abundant world where resources flow easily, you are provided for, and life works out in your favor or as a stingy, deficient world where there is never enough and you have to work hard to just barely get by. *It's a quantum shift that allows what you are seeing and experiencing to be perceived completely differently.* That shift takes place within you.

In the body, the high-vibrational frequency field will emerge as the presence of vibrant, healthy cells, absorption of nutrients taking place easily, detoxification happening smoothly, cells regenerating, and energy flowing and being restored. In this high frequency, the immune system is strong, and we stay healthy no matter what environment we are in. We reside in a reality where the body functions in harmony as it was designed to do.

When we are in fear, the body clamps down into the fight-or-flight, suppressive state of control. The field contracts and registers at a lower frequency. Bodily functions are interrupted, and fear can bring us onto all kinds of paths of animosity. When we welcome rather than reject the animosity, we return to a degree of flow and acceptance. The body relaxes, and the parasympathetic state takes over and changes everything. Our thoughts and beliefs determine the state in which the body resides.

I utilized this truth during my internship year—the first year of my residency training. I had become terribly sick and couldn't go to work. It felt like one of those horrible viral illnesses where I'd be in bed for a few days. I felt into where this was coming from and immediately became aware of something that had happened during my shift the day before. I had been visiting my patient, a young boy who'd been in the rehabilitation unit for a couple of months after a spinal cord injury. As I had leaned over to listen to his heart, he coughed a wet, junky cough—right in my face. As I reviewed the experience, I became aware at that very moment I had been thinking: *Oh no, this is very bad*, and had felt doom and vulnerability.

I brought up that exact moment in my awareness and cleared the fear I had felt. I share a process for how to do this later in this book. I activated my energy and told my body: *I am powerful and resilient. I am healthy and strong.* I saw myself unplugging from the ideas I had previously been holding. Immediately I felt lighter. My body still felt ill, but the heaviness and dread that had been there before were gone. The powerlessness lifted and I felt stronger.

Within a day, I recovered and was back at work. I decided I would remain strong no matter what conditions or people I was exposed to and that my immune system and health were more powerful than any of them. During the remaining three years of my residency and years as an attending physician in Emergency Medicine, having been exposed to thousands of sick patients, I never again became affected this way. I know my resiliency is a direct result of my conscious choice to unplug from the ideas about vulnerability to others and the fear of getting sick.

Beyond just our body, our life circumstances are also positively affected by our high-vibrational state. When we engage in gratitude, acceptance, or self-love, we find life goes more smoothly for us; what might be a problem for others will seem to work out easily, and we'll witness problems dissolve. Creating this shift doesn't even require a huge change within us. It's a quantum shift, a tweak. In fact, just the act of softening the body and breathing more fully can massively change external circumstances.

You may have noticed this in your own life. When you're in a state of flow and well-being, you notice more synchronicities, such as being in the right place at the right time, meeting people who are exactly the right person for a project you're working on, or serendipitously finding a relationship match.

I met my husband this way, in fact. I had suffered greatly in my relationships until, finally, enough was enough. I was in great pain and anguish over a pattern I hadn't been able to see. I decided I would take full responsibility for my relationship outcomes. It wasn't my fault these things had happened, but it was 100% my responsibility to own them and allow them to change.

I began to express gratitude for everything that was showing up instead of complaining about what wasn't. I even went so far as to give thanks for the awesome partner I hadn't yet met. I lay there on my rooftop, looking up at the stars with gratitude for this gift before it showed up. I got into such a high-vibrational state, tears streamed from my eyes, and I felt such a sense of fulfillment and elation, my body shook. Within days I was introduced to my now husband. Yup! A friend who'd known him for years saw him again and instantly knew. She told him, "You've got to call my friend Kim!" and the rest is history. Mario knew within moments of meeting me that I was the one for him.

He told his sister that evening, "I've met the woman I'm going to marry." I knew exactly three weeks later he was my guy. That's how powerful and certain circumstances can be if we allow them to manifest when we first connect with the frequency of our intention and then stay in flow.

When we're in a low-vibrational state—tense, angry, grumpy— there's a space of resistance, and the physical matter—which, remember, is almost all empty space—is going to feel different. There will be constant challenges, hardship, circumstances not working out for us, money being hard to come by, and recurrent relationship disasters.

Our life circumstances will reflect our beliefs, such as:

Life is hard.

I never get what I want.

Only bad things happen to me.

Nothing works out.

If something goes well, the other shoe drops and it all falls apart.

This is because our own frequency and vibration directly affect physical matter. We are not in a physical universe but an electromagnetic field. The consciousness we are in, our thoughts and beliefs, determines the frequency of that field and so determines how life and reality appear. When we see the physical thing, the *stuff*, and think that is the prime reality or the cause, we are missing out on the real leverage, which is the ability to interact with and change reality, sometimes quickly, and transmute it into something higher.

The shift in the physical takes place with even a subtle tweak in the quantum—a slight lightening up or surrender. It's not about turning your liver into a cat. It's about turning a cancerous liver cell into a healthy liver cell. It's a tweak at the quantum level to produce this shift at the physical level. This shift is not far away, not difficult. I show in this book how to do it.

You may make it difficult; you may struggle to "shift your frequency," but I would invite you instead to simply soften. Soften your body and let the breath come slightly more fluidly. That surrender in a moment of intense fear takes great courage. It's not nothing. It's everything. That surrender from fighting, trying, and making it happen is the shift. When you let go, you allow something within you to do the work for you. This is the shift in frequency that will move the planet and change your world.

Limiting beliefs alter your brain function, so you cannot possibly see what is beyond the ideas you hold. Certain perspectives you hold will activate parts of your brain and shut other parts down. There could be tons of money available, amazing opportunities, and ways for your body to easily regain health, but when you hold ideas such as: *It won't work, I can't leave my job, there are no good mates out there,* or *I'll never get better,* you cannot perceive those higher possibilities.

Negative ideas keep generalized inflammation going and put the nervous system into the sympathetic, fight-or-flight state. Your body stays in a stress state, so it cannot heal disease. When your perspective is that the world you've been shown is the only reality available, you limit the kind of possibilities you let in.

For example, if someone diagnosed with Hashimoto's thyroiditis, an autoimmune disorder that causes low thyroid function, thinks: *My thyroid is not working, I have a bad thyroid,* or *I have this disease,* there is detriment to the body. If they continue to hold tight to the perspective that the disease is a separate entity, that their body is purely physical, and that their thyroid is broken, they will not conceive of or perceive solutions that lie beyond this. They will not experience the truth that the energy field they're in could shift to allow their thyroid to be fully healthy and function well.

Their body could shift to stop overtaxing their adrenals and move more into the parasympathetic state—or *relaxation response*—and heal. They might let in the possibility that a medication or a treatment could help them deal with it, but they are still functioning in the reality of: *I have this disease and I have to manage it.* Their brain will not register information outside that, so they will not see those solutions or choose them.

When I was working in the osteopathic clinic during my Osteopathic Medicine Fellowship—a year-long program in which I received extra training in how to support the body in healing itself—I noticed that patients who identified with their diagnoses were often more resistant to healing. Patients would say things like: *I know you can't heal my fibromyalgia, but maybe you can help make it more livable,* or they'd say: *They already did the labs, and my thyroid doesn't work, so I'll always need medication.*

Those patients would continue to decline, and the effort to help them was exhausting. The more they bought into the *reality* of their diagnosis and everything they believed it to mean, the more difficult it would be to assist them with healing. However, when there was no clear diagnosis or when the patient didn't believe the diagnosis was true, it actually helped. Outcomes were different when the patient wasn't holding firm beliefs or conclusions about what was happening in their body.

One patient I worked with had been diagnosed with multiple sclerosis (MS). She had also been told she had chronic fatigue syndrome. Over the years, her condition had progressively become worse, and she was losing her ability to walk. She found out about my work and wondered if it could help her. She had been told by multiple doctors that her condition would continue to worsen. She had been put on a trial of a new medication but had not seen significant results. We met online for virtual sessions, and she told me: *They say I have MS, but I don't think that's what's going on.*

She wondered if there was a way her body could reverse her inflammatory symptoms. She was open; she was curious. She was willing to consider something outside what she had been told was true. Over time, working together in what is now my Embracing Health program, we found she had repressed feelings of sadness and abandonment from her childhood, having been raised with lots of siblings, feeling like there wasn't enough love to go around. She recognized patterns of suppressing her own needs and pretending to be happy as a survival mechanism.

This patient saw patterns in her life of withholding her feelings, not because she didn't want to be open with her husband and family but because she'd never considered it would do any good to share her feelings. She had learned they were inconvenient and didn't matter, so she had learned to shut them out. Her body suffered. She became aware that she had been on an autopilot program, doing for others and giving to everyone else but leaving herself out of the equation entirely. At first, she became angry about this and had a sense of powerlessness, as if no matter what she did, she would never retrieve her sense of self and ability to express her needs.

In the Embracing Health group, we used the MindBody healing work to resolve the belief systems and unconscious programming that had kept her stuck and kept her emotions repressed. She was able to release the past patterns from her nervous system so she could now register her own emotions, ask for what she needed, and be willing to receive from others who loved her. This changed the state of her nervous system. She was no longer being that false-self, the one who was created to cope with her earlier situation.

She regained her motor function. Fatigue resolved and her energy returned. Over the next several months, she started walking again. She resumed golfing with her husband and was able to participate in family activities. Because she had opened up to the possibility her body could shift out of the pattern the doctors were calling MS, she was able to create a healthy life. She even found this experience and what it called her to confront had greatly improved her family life and relationships.

Another patient I worked with, Karen, was a medical student. Karen had been diagnosed with Hashimoto's thyroid disease, anxiety disorder, and chronic fatigue syndrome. An ultrasound had demonstrated nodules on her thyroid, and her labs revealed that her thyroid function was low. Doctors told her she would require medications for life and possibly thyroid surgery.

When we did the MindBody work together, we uncovered a pattern in Karen of shutting out her body's messages. Karen would push through fatigue and work hard to study and achieve. When she became fatigued, she used energy drinks and pushed herself harder. She gained weight and felt powerless over her body. She tried to increase her running to get her energy up and control her weight. Karen developed pain in her body and more severe fatigue until she was no longer able to run. Her condition deteriorated, and she felt there was nothing she could do to fight this.

Together we uncovered her huge amount of judgment of her body, her fear of gaining weight and losing control of her body, and her resentment in the relationship with her mother. This last part is something almost always present when women have eating disorders, weight problems, or issues with food. Karen also became aware of a fear of inadequacy and failure. This was evidenced by patterns of constantly pushing herself harder and having low grades at school, to the point of nearly failing out of medical school. We uncovered patterns in her relationships of denying her feelings and going along with what her partner wanted. She had little sexual desire and thought something was wrong with her. She pretended to be someone she was not to make her relationships work.

As we deepened her sense of connection and presence in her body, Karen released anger, fear, and self-doubt and was able to resolve the resentment toward her mother. She expressed her true feelings in her relationship and honored her emotions. She released the fear of failure and stopped pushing herself. She was able to slow down when she needed rest and found her body would reboot itself within a short time when she did. She was able to enjoy running again without pain.

Within a couple of months, Karen's energy returned and her weight came back to normal. When her labs and ultrasound were rechecked, her thyroid function was normal and there were no more thyroid nodules.

Had the problem been coming from Karen's thyroid, or was her body's energy so depleted from trying to run the false programs that the thyroid lacked the capacity to do its job?

When Karen could again access all the energy that had been used to suppress emotions and feed the false-self, her body could restore and heal. Had she bought into the idea of thyroid disease as a condition to fight against or manage for life, she may not have opened to allowing a more expansive approach. Because she was able to allow a massive shift in her consciousness and let go of the false-self, her body healed very quickly, and the physical signs of illness reversed.

To experience a quantum shift like Karen's, allow a shift in your perspective. Be open to a higher possibility. Realize you are pure energy, not just physical. When you understand you are pure energy, it's easier to imagine a small shift can allow your chemistry to change, your hormones to rebalance, and your thyroid, adrenals, immune system, and digestive system to have all the energy they need to regain full function and health.

The physical body reflects the energy template. The body is just showing us what we're holding. It's reflecting the resistance held in our system that's ready to go. Lovingly acknowledging that we're in resistance is enough. Find compassion for the one within who is too scared to let go or who doesn't know how. That's enough. Remember, a small quantum shift equals big physical changes.

No disease is more powerful than the power
within you to generate change.

You will not receive and experience anything that you do not allow yourself first to perceive and consider. You must first open before the new experience can come in.

Are you willing to suspend disbelief, let go of control, and be guided from a space that is higher than what you have imagined yourself to be?

This quantum rearrangement also applies to our relationships. If you have thoughts about people in your life like: *He is a narcissist*, or *She is selfish*, they directly impact the way you see that person. Even if that person has the ability to be kind, loving, compassionate, and self-reflective, you will not have that experience of them. Even if they were to be incredibly conscious, they would not appear differently for you because you are holding your perceptions of them so strongly.

Others are directly impacted by the thoughts and conclusions you hold about them. Whether or not they know it consciously, your energy is impacting them. Your body emits an electromagnetic field felt by others around you. A person feels your judgment, resentment, and anger, which affects their cellular function, brain function, thoughts, and behavior.

Unless they are very conscious, they remain in the same pattern you are holding them in. Even if they behave differently around others and could access a kinder, more evolved way of being, this is less likely to happen when they are in a field of judgment and negativity.

This is how *our perspective equals our reality*. We emit that perspective as a field of energy out to the world. When we maintain the perspective: *life is hard*, it shows up that way. When we embrace the idea: *I'm powerful in ways I hadn't imagined*, or even just the openness of: *I wonder how things might be different for me*, possibilities open up. When we see the world as only solid and physical, we are limited in what possibilities show up in our lives. We don't realize that we, through our very thoughts, are having an impact on everything around us.

One woman I worked with shared in our group about challenges with her husband. She stated this approach didn't apply to her because her husband would never change and didn't have the capacity to feel anything. "My husband is a narcissist," she explained. "I can't have a better relationship, so I have to make do with what I've got."

I suspected there were some strong conclusions she was holding that kept the situation from shifting, so I asked if she was open to a new perspective.

"Yes," she said eagerly. "I would love that!"

I asked her to consider the possibility her own energy field could be keeping her from experiencing something new with him, and perhaps there could be more possible in her relationship with her husband. "You're only seeing the aspect of him that shows up in the energy field you are currently residing in. Who knows what's possible when you shift your energy?"

Months later she told me, "I never would have believed it could happen, but I kept applying this work, kept softening to let go of my perspective, and stayed open. I let go of tension and frustration, and I let go of the ideas about him and stayed curious instead. One morning when he came into the kitchen, I said 'Good morning!' in my usual cheerful way, and he scoffed, 'What's so good about it?' I got so mad and felt my body harden. Then I decided maybe I could soften and just feel the moment and let the energy move through. As I breathed, it occurred to me to touch him gently and ask him what he needed. It was so unexpected. He turned to me and said, 'I need to feel you. I need you to be real with me.' He explained that when I'm so cheerful, he gets the sense that I'm faking it, that I'm not present, and he can't feel my joy. It never occurred to me that he wanted to feel me."

When *you* shift, you create space for something deeper in others. You are not the reason someone is abusing you, and you don't need to stay in an abusive relationship and keep trying to change yourself. Often, when you make a shift in consciousness, one of the most powerful things that can happen is you are easily able to exit a relationship when you previously saw no options.

Whether you are dealing with a *narcissistic husband*, an *overbearing mother*, a *difficult child*, or anyone who seems impossible, check in to see what energies you may be unconsciously holding on to keeping you in that experience.

I've witnessed unthinkable changes happen in relationships with children and loved ones in my Embracing Health course. No matter how stuck something may seem, soften to let the energy go, and then see what is possible. This especially applies to abusive relationships you just can't seem to get out of. You're sucked back into the dynamic over and over and don't have the resources to leave. When you *shift your energy* first, you will go from having no solutions and feeling stuck to seeing the doors open and having full confidence and clarity to walk away. Always honor your safety. Do not allow yourself to remain in situations where you are being harmed. Shift within, and you *will* see the way out.

One woman in my Embracing Health group shared that her adopted teenage child had been struggling with severe suicidality for years, and the situation had overtaken their whole family. They lived in constant fear and stress, trying to care for this child who refused to accept their help and was exhibiting very destructive behaviors. She was at her wit's end, and they had finally institutionalized the child.

We focused on releasing the fear in this mother's body. She had fully let in all her deepest fears as well as the guilt she had been holding. With deep compassion, she let go of the fight-or-flight state she had been in for years with her family and this child. After doing this work and witnessing the profound emotions she had been holding, she felt freer, lighter. In the following group call, she reported a massive change in her daughter's behavior: she communicated with the family and let them in, her destructive behavior changed, and she was no longer suicidal.

Your system is involved in the energies of everything and everyone you experience. This type of shift could never be done through blaming yourself for someone else's destructive behavior. You must take full responsibility for your experience *and* be willing to embrace what is here as it is.

A major step is letting go of the problem as a solid thing that cannot be changed. Once we let go, emotions arise that can be released. It was challenging for this mother to embrace the enormity of her fear and guilt, but when she was willing to do this, she set it free.

The same goes for an illness. When you own a disease as a physical entity, *my fibromyalgia*, you are creating a reality in which the disease or the situation has power. You give it power—unconsciously, of course. You are creating the circumstance that causes your body to align with low energy or intense pain or a feeling of powerlessness, so solutions do not appear. With compassion, you can witness this and allow a shift. Compassion is key, though; you must let go of making yourself wrong. You didn't really have a choice until now.

Many patients have said to me, "I have seen so many doctors for this, but they have all failed me." This is what happens when we are living in the perception that illness is happening to us: *Nothing works. No one can help me*, they say. That is powerlessness. It will keep happening again and again until you shift at that level. To do this requires great compassion for the one inside who has suffered. You cannot make yourself wrong for feeling like a victim or being a victim. You are not at fault for anything that has happened in your past. You are, however, given the opportunity to take full responsibility for everything that happens from here forward. This is the stance we take when we are truly ready for change.

> *Reality exists only where the mind creates a focus.*
> ~Mahayana Buddhism Sutra

Where is your focus when you perceive your illness, symptom, person, or problem? Is it on freedom and peace, or fear?

> *We are reality makers, and we create*
> *what we believe in our hearts.*
> ~ Gregg Braden

You are not at fault. You *are* responsible.

CHAPTER TWO

You Are a Creator

YOUR EXPERIENCES ARE DETERMINED BY YOUR CONSCIOUSNESS

Our actions, behaviors, and even our voices carry the vibration of our inner consciousness. Our consciousness impacts everything and changes everything in our lives. Let's look at an example of how subtle changes in our inner consciousness can lead to major changes in our outer life circumstance. Say you are standing in line for coffee and you are keeping to yourself, not looking around, not smiling or being particularly friendly. You purchase your coffee, get in your car, and go about your day.

Now let's say there is 2% more lightness within you, 2% more softening, and 2% more full breath. You are standing in line, feeling slightly more uplifted than you would have been. You look up and smile at the person beside you and let out a big exhale, softening your body more fully. That person senses you and exhales as well. You each say hello and start up a brief conversation. You find out they are an amazing healer who has the exact solution to everything you are dealing with right now. The solution is easy and something you can implement right away. Or let's say that person is looking for someone who does exactly the work you do and is looking to hire or collaborate with someone just like you. Or maybe they say something so funny, you start cracking up and your mood is uplifted for the entire day. This exchange powerfully changes the trajectory of your day, your choices and behaviors, and, potentially, your entire life. Your life can shift its trajectory like this in any given moment.

How you show up in each moment is determined by your consciousness. It is determined by your electromagnetics. The electromagnetic signals emanating from your body allow for possibilities, synchronicities, and chance meetings you could never have planned. They can create a path of healing, the path of your ideal relationships, or a path of amazing opportunities in your work and money. Maybe a brilliant idea that changes the course of your life sparks in your mind. You have all the energy and inspiration to put it into action, and you are never the same. Any moment can be a moment of great inspiration that allows your life to enter a new trajectory.

Every moment contains a choice: to open or to close. Opening takes courage, compassion, and a willingness to play along. We not only feel lighter and ignite the parasympathetic nervous system that restores health, but we also enter a higher vibrational state that changes our thoughts, actions, and behaviors. Closing can feel temporarily protective and give you moments of escape, but that feeling will not last, and it shuts down possibilities. Through reading this book, you will learn the value of staying open and receptive. You will gain the ability to do so no matter what may be going on. You will develop the awareness needed to choose receptivity again and again, so you access infinite power and allow instant healing.

We will see synchronicities and serendipities arise when we generate a high-vibrational frequency. Life flows effortlessly. The electromagnetics in a lower frequency, however, create the opposite. In this case, nothing ever goes right for you. You work hard to make things happen and money is still limited. Your energy is low, and you never get what you want. Lower-frequency energy will play out the script that you have embodied in your perception. Typically, these circumstances cause us to close even further into fight-or-flight, clamping down into efforting. This activates the sympathetic nervous system and leads to fast, shallow breathing, tension in the body, and brain patterns that run our limiting beliefs on a loop.

We therefore don't see possibility and don't understand how things could be different. We double down on tension and control, trying harder to muscle through our moment. We do this, of course, until it's clear it won't work, and until it creates more and more pain and lack. And then, finally, we surrender and allow some opening. We let go of trying, the body softens, and our breath begins to deepen. That's the moment when things can finally change.

Every moment, including this one right now,
contains the seed for potent change.

Program or Truth: Seeing Through the Illusion

If unconscious programs are running the show, triggering our systems to close off to our Life Force, putting us into chronic fight-or-flight mode and limiting our health and prosperity, where do these patterns come from, and how do they become so embedded?

Why don't we notice ourselves making the choice to close?

The subconscious closure patterns are automatic and result from our brain functioning and neural networks. Once we run a program of thought/emotion/reaction, as Canadian neuropsychologist Donald Hebb coined in 1949, "neurons that fire together, wire together." That pattern strengthens the pathways of those thoughts, those emotions, and those reactions. We think: *It's just who I am* or *who someone else is.*

We may say: *I'm shy in social situations,* or *He's an angry person.*

This becomes what I call the *protective personality*. The protective personality is the sum total of all the habits, beliefs, conclusions, assumptions, and behaviors that stem from our past memories, traumas, suppressed emotions, and limited experiences. The protective personality runs the program of closure, tension, and inflammation, as well as the behaviors that shut out love, resources, and opportunities. When we live from the protective personality—a form of the small-self—life will seem limited because it is reflecting our limited self.

At any one time your health is the sum total of all the impulses, positive and negative, emanating from your consciousness.
~ Deepak Chopra

I want to make a quick note about trauma. Extensive research demonstrates the link between childhood trauma and adult-onset chronic illness. I've worked with many adults with chronic illnesses who have clear, identifiable trauma in their past, and I have also worked with many adults with chronic illnesses who have been unable to pinpoint any major traumas. We don't need to have had what we consider a significant incident to incorporate these patterns of closure, tension, inflammation, and chronic illness.

Just the experience of being raised in a society that tells you, "Your power is outside yourself," and "Your value is conditional" is traumatic to an awakened being.

The good news is you don't need to find the trauma, and you certainly don't need to re-live it. You just need to feel into the *now*. The programming that's active in your system here, now. Let go of searching your past, and let go of needing a reason to validate negative emotions by finding an identifiable cause. You were fed falsehoods about yourself and about your value. That alone is enough to instill the kind of closure and chronic fight-or-flight living that can cause massive problems in adulthood.

I also want to say that the Source Consciousness that created you can also allow major healing within you, no matter how severe or ingrained the traumas you may have lived through may be.

Do not think: *My trauma is too big; this will take longer,* or *My problem has been going on for many years, so I'll never be free.* It's not true. Yes, you may have more reasons to clamp down and identify as the small-self, but you are free to release them whenever you are ready. I've witnessed people heal massive traumas within minutes. Trauma can arrive within minutes, so why wouldn't it be able to leave within minutes? It's just programming; it only has the power you give it. Give yourself space around trauma and lots of compassion.

Suppressed Emotions Keep You Stuck

Our emotions activate a particular brain state—a particular neurologic pattern—and they are meant to move through us, not be suppressed. When we are in a state of anger or fear, the brain functions in a limited way. We see only the short-term need for escape, relief, or immediate gratification. This is meant to be a survival mechanism, but most of the emotions that arise, as intense as they may be, are not indicators of a true threat. They result from a perceived threat, but they register in the body as if we are truly threatened. We feel sadness, shame, and loneliness, and those feelings trigger us to eat cake, for example, so we feel the sweetness of life again. When we suppress emotions and live in chronic fight-or-flight, the nervous system stays turned on, as if we are under survival threat. The brain looks for the immediate solution. It clamps down into single-minded focus.

We no longer see the big picture; we only see the beliefs and perspectives that are wired into that emotional state. The brain says: *Get me out of here!* or *Fix this!* and automated behaviors kick in. We behave unconsciously and robotically at that point. The program runs us, and we don't even question what is happening. This is what happens when we close. We clamp down to *control*. We don't feel. We don't recognize that we ourselves are restricting the Life Force, the healing, the infinite possibilities that are flowing toward us. The protective personality runs the program of closure. Eventually, we see no way to do otherwise. We think: *I have to do this. That's life.*

If we instead *open*—soften the body, deepen the breath—we allow our emotions to flow fluidly. The underlying energy of anger or fear can release within seconds. We can have a whole different experience of the moment, beyond what the pattern says is true. We bend "reality" because we enter a more harmonious state of being. This is a state of *nonresistance*, and it allows the body to function in resilience and flow.

Most of us do not do this. We have learned to habitually suppress our emotions and haven't learned how to discharge anger, fear, or other challenging emotions. Most of us have resistance to the lower emotions, so we act out in unhealthy ways, trying to protect ourselves from our own feelings, or we suppress our emotions to numb ourselves. Science has demonstrated the toxic effects of this and how anger, fear, and shame suppress the healthy functioning of the body. They bring us into a lower electromagnetic frequency, a more inflamed and disruptive chemistry, and a more limiting physiologic functioning. This suppressive state is not one of ease; it's *dis-ease*.

The lower emotions themselves are not harmful. It's *resistance* to the lower emotions that generates inflammation, disease, adrenal fatigue, cancer, autoimmunity (the body attacking itself), and depletion of the health. *Emotions are energy in motion*. The energy wants to move. It's meant to move through us. When we hold resistance, energy is suppressed. The energy resurfaces only when we're overloaded and can't suppress it anymore. Emotion arises in overwhelming bursts when we're triggered or when we just can't keep it all in any longer. We may see these moments as a weakness because we've been led to believe that being emotional—expressing our emotional energy and letting it be seen—is wrong. Indeed, many authoritarian institutional structures have taught this. That's because people cannot be controlled and manipulated when they allow their energy and emotions to move freely.

Welcoming and expressing your emotions will bring change. Outer authoritarian structures vested in you staying the same won't like that—but it will free *you* and, ultimately, those structures as well. It is healthy to honor, respect, and *express* emotions. When we subscribe to authoritarian programming that says we should be obedient, do as we're told, and not to think for ourselves, we obey the rules of that program and are unhealthy. We are under its control. The tension and resistance of suppressed emotions become chronic and affect brain function, limiting everything we do, think, and see.

When you are under the control of the programming, your brain will reflect the truth of the B.S. (a.k.a. Belief Systems) of that programming. For example, if you believe: *I will never make it,* or *I am not good enough,* or: *All of this stuff I'm reading is crap, it won't work for me,* it fires off all the neurons in your brain that carry evidence of all the times when you failed or when things did not work out. You ignite all the memories that prove you right, all the times you were taken advantage of, all the times you were not good enough, all the times you were inadequate—even if that's not what actually happened. In fact, your brain is very good at fabricating evidence of false memories. It makes stuff up. Your brain will mirror your beliefs, and you will think: *I'm right!*

One of my greatest teachers asked me during a workshop, "Would you rather be right or be happy?" It was a choice I had to make. My brain really wanted to be right, but in that moment I witnessed all it was costing me to keep doing so.

My life was misery, and there was no joy. A part of me—the ego—didn't like this insight and wanted to keep being right about being miserable. Thankfully, though, I got it. I chose to let go of being right. I chose to let go of seeing things the way I was seeing them. I chose to let go of my own perception and be open to something higher.

What do you choose?

Changing Your Pattern of Being

You can change the pattern of being the protective personality, the small-self, by altering your inner state. You can move from closure—tension, control, fight-or-flight—to opening—softness, receptivity, slow breath. It's a quantum shift within you that allows the outer, seemingly static circumstances to shift. Remember that whatever is happening is okay.

Say to yourself: *It's okay to feel this. It's okay to let this in. I accept myself and my moment fully.*

Doing so activates the part of your brain with memories of things that *did* work out for you, times when you were courageous and when things went smoothly. You begin to realize you are capable, life is on your side, and it *is* okay to make choices that allow expansion in your life.

The change can sometimes happen very quickly. Once we get into a more receptive state, we're more aware of our heart's calling and inner inspiration. We have clarity where there was previously confusion. We have an insight where previously we were blank. We feel moved to take a certain action when previously we had been apathetic.

Suppose you have a spontaneous idea to call your friend. You do not know where that idea came from, but you act and synchronicity happens. Your friend tells you, "I was thinking about you. I have this amazing opportunity for you," and something prosperous comes out of that phone call, or you have a feeling of lightness after the call that wouldn't have been there before.

> *The moment you stand in agreement to the moment*
> *you stand in is the only place God can be found.*
> ~ Paul Selig

Are you open to more moments like that?

When we embrace a more open emotional state, we are in a higher electromagnetic frequency, causing the brain to perceive little bits of intuition that will lead to a favorable outcome in our lives.

I worked with one client who made a huge shift in her inner perspective and released lots of old suppressed emotions in her system. The very next day, she spontaneously found the exact homeopathic remedy that resolved her unrelenting hyperthyroid disease. She had been in and out of the hospital with severe symptoms for years due to *thyroid storm*, wherein the thyroid is overactive and puts the body into a crisis state. It can be life-threatening. She had tried everything, and then the day after our session in which we shifted the underlying energies, she was able to find this resolution. That's the needle-in-a-haystack moment. You can't try to make that happen. You can only surrender to allow what is ready to take place for you.

If you stay open to your moment and allow a more fluid emotional state—a higher frequency—you access all those powerful occurrences and allow magical things to happen. Your mind-body system can function in a way that lets those miraculous synchronicities occur easily. It's not *you* doing it. Life Force is coming through you to create it. There's an infinite difference.

What You Resist Persists: Why Fighting Disease Can't Create Health

As a physician, I have witnessed an avid societal focus on fighting disease. There's the *war against cancer*. We are going to *fight diabetes* and *combat obesity*. We are not appreciating the fact that the fight state (part of the fight-or-flight nervous system) creates an autoimmune inflammatory response when we reside in it all the time. That survival mechanism serves us in the short term should we ever have to outrun the tiger or find the highest tree to get out of trouble. However, we must promptly return to the rest-and-digest stage, the restoration state after a burst of activity.

Returning to the restoration state—the relaxation response—does not happen easily in our society right now. We can be in a constant state of fight-or-flight from watching the news or from constant worry about finances or relationships. You have been taught to constantly control your body, control your weight, fight your disease, or wage a war on your cancer.

How is it going?

That approach works dynamically against everything you are intending. The sympathetic nervous system—the fight, flight, or freeze response—was not designed to work for extended periods of time. Being in this state for hours or days on end will create inflammation throughout the entire body. It is going to increase stress, increase cortisol—the main stress hormone— and other inflammatory hormones. Your body begins to function in dis-ease—not the ease and flow and harmony that lets the body heal and restore itself. In this inflamed state, the body cannot do its general housekeeping: releasing waste products, digesting your food, absorbing nutrients, and detoxifying. All of that gets turned off in the fight-or-flight state.

You cannot be in a relaxed state of restoration—taking in nutrients that support the body, repairing and detoxifying the body— when you are in the fight-or-flight state. That will all get put aside, and you'll end up living in a chronic state of tension. There will be pain in the muscles that will not resolve because there is not enough relaxation to allow energy to move, letting in oxygen and nutrients and moving out waste products. Gut and stomach problems arise, so it becomes impossible to digest even the most basic food, and a strict diet becomes necessary. Inflammation can arise throughout the bowel and gut that will be diagnosed as Crohn's disease, or the ulcerative colitis or inflammatory bowel disease I lived with. On the surface, that will seem to be the problem, but it's only a reflection of the underlying imbalance in the system.

We think these symptoms are a force in and of themselves, but they are indicators the body is responding to the state of consciousness we are in. As soon as we start trying to *fight* disease, we are in a stress state. The fighting mindset engages an inner state that inhibits health, shuts off the restorative housekeeping processes of the parasympathetic nervous system, and prevents our body from working as it was designed to. *Para* means around, and the para-sympathetic nervous system is located *around* the sympathetic nervous system. The sympathetic nerves reside in the thoracic area, the torso. Parasympathetic nerves are above and below the torso, thus *around* the sympathetic nervous system, in the cranial and sacral areas of the body—the head and the bottom.

This is one reason why craniosacral work can be so powerful; it activates the parasympathetic nervous system, which is the opposite of the fight-flight-freeze response. The parasympathetic nervous system ignites the relaxation response. Understanding this is a major key to unlocking the conundrum of so many diseases in the mainstream perspective. Although there has been extensive research for decades, it has not been integrated into mainstream institutional medical education or practice.

Herbert Benson's book *The Relaxation Response*, first published in 1976, documents decades of research and many ways the parasympathetic, relaxation response is healing to the body. This part of the involuntary nervous system, when active, enhances detoxification, strengthens immune function, enhances blood flow and cellular regeneration, and improves brain and nervous system functioning. It also decreases inflammation—which is the underlying physiology for every major fatal disease like heart disease, obesity, cancer, and diabetes—and it allows the body to heal itself.

When you remember the relaxation response is incredibly powerful, encompasses *every* level of healing, and activates your inner wisdom that *does* know how to reverse the disease even when your healthcare team doesn't, you find the willingness to surrender. You allow your body to reside in a parasympathetic state more fully. The parasympathetic state is activated when you are in a higher vibrational state of self-acceptance and self-love. It allows you to immediately reverse disease and strengthen the body.

It can be hard to imagine not fighting your disease when you think the disease is more powerful than you are. You've been taught disease is an entity with a life of its own, so, of course, you think you think you need to fight against it. Maybe you fear if you stop fighting, you will succumb and the disease will win. You may fear if you don't fight your fatigue, you'll become a blob on the couch who never leaves the house. I know I did. I was terrified of surrender.

Let's get clear on what has been created with the *fight* approach, which is also recognized as the small-self-trying-to-heal-myself approach. You've probably lived in some level of fight-or-flight much of your life.

Ask yourself:

What gets created when my small-self is in tension, control, and fight?

Has it led to greater health, well-being, freedom, and vitality?

Or has it led to more diagnoses, more complex problems, more challenges and overwhelm, and more compounding fatigue?

Noticing this is powerful! I welcome you to share your insights with this and any other experiences while reading this book with the MindBody Community on Facebook, found at https://www.facebook.com/groups/mindbodycommunity. For pretty much everyone I work with, the latter is the rule; it is what has been their reality. And no matter how many problems or diagnoses they may have, there is one antidote: It takes surrender. *If I stop fighting and let go, the wisdom in my body can take over and something can happen for me.*

I invite you to release the idea that health comes *from* you, that you have to fight for it, and that you have to make it happen. Instead, embrace the idea that health comes *through* you. The more you are in surrender, relaxation, and allowing, the more powerfully health, Life Force, comes into your cells to return them to a balanced state.

It takes a little bit of courage at first to surrender, soften, and breathe deeply while facing a perceived threat. However, if you are willing to be curious and suspend doubt as you read this book, you allow that activation within you so that health comes through you. You let the Intelligence that created you flow through you more fully and create all those results you have been fighting so hard to get.

> *As below, so above, and as above, so below.*
> *With this knowledge alone you may work miracles.*
> ~ The Emerald Tablet

LIFE COMES THROUGH YOU, NOT FROM YOU

To tap infinite power for instant healing, you must stop seeing yourself as primarily physical. As long as you see yourself as a separate physical entity, you will continue to fight illness and fight against life. When you understand you are the Consciousness observing it all and your body is pure energy, you let in a new realm of possibility. You understand life is not happening to you; the disease is not happening to you; something within your energy field has created it. Past childhood trauma is linked to adult chronic illness, anxiety, and depression, but don't try to get rid of the trauma or heal the trauma. That can't be done because what you focus on expands. When you try to heal the trauma, your focus is on the trauma. As you get better at fixing it, it gets better at existing. This is exactly what happened to me when I was sick with an autoimmune disease. I kept trying to heal myself. I kept trying to heal my illness. I understood something in me created it, but I was so identified with that self, I thought *I* created it. I thought: *I can fix this.* It was an illusion.

Let Go of Trying to Manifest Health

When we think: *Okay, if I created this, I can fix it,* we are still living in separation. We are still living in fear and lack. We are still coming from the perspective that *we* are the physical, solid separate self. We are still identifying as the small-self. That's why nothing works. The small-self has no power. This is not because it's wrong or bad or unwanted. It's because the small-self is invented. The small-self isn't *real*.

Who are you?

You are not your body. You are the Consciousness observing all of this.

If you were to lose an arm, an ear, or another body part, you would still exist, wouldn't you? If you had a traumatic experience that changed your life, you would still exist even if you were to let go and heal that trauma, would you not?

If I were to ask who are you, and you think: *I'm a mother*, or *I'm a caretaker*, or *I'm a lawyer*, are you still that person even if the relationship ends or the job goes away? If emotions come and go and thoughts come and go, are you your thoughts and emotions? If you are not your body, you are not your roles, and you are not your experiences and feelings, who are you?

Hmm.

You are the space and Consciousness observing all of this. You are part of the *Creator*, not the created. You are not the small-self. It's a fabrication. When you identify as the small-self—a congregate of personality traits, illnesses, experiences, roles—you lock yourself into powerlessness and limitation. That's not because you're bad, wrong, or unworthy; it's because the small-self doesn't exist.

Do you see how we can use this to beat ourselves down and prove to ourselves that we really are powerless and limited?

Everything you see as solid is pure energy. Your external conditions that seem stuck and impossible to change are pure energy. The body and its ailments and symptoms are just pure energy. All the matter in the Universe is impacted by the field of energy it is within. *You* are a field of energy. You can change matter. You can change your body. You must start by letting go of who and what you think you are.

The Intelligence that created everything created you and your liver, kidneys, and digestive system—all of your body. This Intelligence is still present and is coursing through you right now. You are still connected with it, and healing with Intelligence is a matter of opening to that more fully and letting it in to rearrange things. The circumstances that have led to the state of disease, no matter how severe, are just a result of the closure where you've restricted that flow.

By surrendering to the fear, hurt, pain, and all the elements that created the closure and tension, you can allow more opening, more softness in your body, so the energy that created you can course through you more freely.

What if that could make all the difference and allow health to be restored? Healing is about allowing and receiving. It is about surrendering rather than trying to manifest and attract or to *make it happen* and *go get it*. That approach may at first be empowering, but eventually it creates tension, inflammation, and all of the fight-or-flight physiology we have talked about.

That is the small-self going to battle. The small-self can't win. It can't do anything. It doesn't exist. You've got to remember you are the Self—capital S—the *I AM Self* or the *Consciousness* observing all. Many different paths can point you to that which you are, but they can't really be understood from a closed mind. They can only be embraced by the heart. However, whether or not you believe this, the truth is the Truth. You—the small-self you—will never create anything. When you surrender, soften, breathe, it activates the *I AM Self*, and then true healing occurs. It's how you are designed.

Everything You Want Is Already Here; Are *You*?

Sit for a moment and ponder these ideas:

- *By letting go, so much more can happen for me.*

- *By allowing even a slightly deeper surrender—2% more softness and openness—I allow more health to course through me and rearrange everything on my behalf: my immune system, my digestion, my nervous system, and my well-being.*

- *What if, just by softening and breathing, everything my heart is asking for could happen for me?*

Notice how you feel. Take a few breaths. Close your eyes. Soften your shoulders. If you registered any sense of lightness, ease, or relaxation, it is because those statements are resonating within you. All we are doing here is allowing you to connect with the truth that already lives in you.

Most people I see are trying to create their health, to fix their health, to whip themselves into shape. They are searching for the right practitioner. They don't want to sit around and do nothing, and that is commendable. They care. They want to be proactive and generate change, but they are going about it from a consciousness of fear, lack, and separation. They are going about it from the small-self who is completely powerless. I've also seen people try to create a more powerful self. They get motivated, more disciplined, more spiritual. They overcome the smallness and are now identifying with a bigger *self*. Great. Yay! It's an exercise. It's something to do. It's not true healing, though. Eventually that diet becomes exhausting, those supplement regimens become too rigid, those intense meditations become too much work, and trying to become a more powerful self is just too much.

From the standpoint of your small-self who has created a personality, you cannot create true health. You create more work, which creates more stress physiology and more wear and tear on the body with fight-or-flight. You work against your intention when you approach it as though the small-self who is creating it.

Try this on instead . . .

Say to yourself:

The Source Consciousness, the Intelligence that created my being, my body, every part in it, every cell, and the way they are interacting and communicating together in every moment, is still here in me right now.

I do not have to create the healing in my body. I do not have to create the circumstances allowing healing to come about.

By allowing 2% more surrender, more relaxation, and more softening, I am more connected with Source Intelligence, and I allow more Source Intelligence to course through me and do what it is designed to do.

I can let go.

Letting go is always going to be a more joyful fluid state than clamping down in fear and tension, trying to control your outcome.

Receive or Resist: You Choose

Now that you understand you are connected to the Source Intelligence that created you, you have a choice. You can open more fully to it, or you can go into further closure. Closure is the inner shutdown and outer tension that causes the fight-flight-or-freeze response to be held excessively. You may have one mode of closure that is most familiar to you.

Closure can be sneaky. Most of us have learned to see our closure patterns as a necessary way of navigating the world, and we do not realize the immense destruction they create. Everything our heart desires would come to us were it not for our closure. All our suffering, lack, and scarcity are direct results of our own closure patterns. Again, these patterns may seem natural to you, or you may think: *I have to do this to survive*—but I'm telling you they are destroying everything most precious to you and keeping all the lack and scarcity in place.

If you knew that behind the door of your own surrender and opening lay everything your Self truly yearns for, would you be more willing to question your closure patterns and consider releasing them?

See if you notice yourself in one or all these patterns of closure. Three main types of closure patterns come from our programming.

1. Fight

    When we're in fight mode, we get defensive, critical of others and ourselves, and feel a need to explain ourselves or our viewpoint to make sure others understand. We focus a lot of mental energy on figuring things out. We feel a need to control our environment. We tend to overcome, achieve, excel, or prove wrong those who said we'd never make it. We are righteous. We think: *I'll show them!* and try to improve ourselves or rise above circumstances and perceived limitations. We try never to let anything get us down and always to do whatever we can to make things right.

    When we're in fight mode, *overwhelm* is the rule.

2. Flight

    When we're in flight mode, we are busy; we *go, go, go!* We talk fast, act fast; we're reactive. We have a hard time slowing down and feel if we do, we will fall behind, lose out, or get into trouble. We may be slow to trust but quick to leave a relationship. We have a pattern of doing many things at once and never feeling satisfied. We're trying to outrun something bad that is about to happen.

    When in flight mode, *insecurity* is the rule.

3. Freeze

    When we go into the freeze pattern, we feel like a powerless victim either to other people, to our illness, or to the conditions of our lives. It seems nothing we do is ever enough. We'll try harder and harder to make our lives work—we care so deeply and give everything of ourselves, but we never seem to have enough time, enough energy, or enough money.

When we're in freeze mode, *lack* is the rule.

It can be helpful to recognize the closure pattern you are in. To the mind, these are going to be patterns that seem necessary and justifiable and possibly patterns the mind can't imagine surviving without.

You close down unconsciously when you get triggered by something someone says or by a memory or circumstance that arises in your life. You do this because you learned it was necessary; then it became an autopilot program. There may have been many times in the past when you weren't capable of managing what was going on, when you were attacked and had to defend, or when you were neglected and had to fend for yourself. You learned to close down and tense your body. You learned certain behaviors for survival.

Maybe that was a good idea in the moment because you were not safe or did not have the resources to process the situation. Maybe it was wise to run, to fight, or to freeze and hold tension to protect yourself from what was taking place. Maybe it was right to suppress your emotions for the time being. Give yourself compassion that you are completely amazing, and it was really smart and wise to do this at that time. It's just not wise to keep doing it now.

By looking at what is true now, which takes immense compassion for the part of you in fear or pain, you can open to a new reality. Start by softening and being tender with yourself, and then get curious and ask: *What is possible now?*

You may notice you're living in closure, unconsciously using the same defense mechanism now, even though you are no longer in an unsafe situation. Realize you are now fully capable of making the choices that keep you safe, or welcoming and expressing emotions so the energy can release. You are provided for now and can do things a different way. You may be conditioned to close from past traumas or a lifetime of fear. You may notice this happening on autopilot. Don't worry. If you stay aware, soften, and breathe into your body, the ability to choose differently will present itself.

You always have the choice, from wherever you are, to reopen.

In fact, as a favorite mentor, Londin Angel Winters, shares, the only two things you have true governance over are where you put your attention and what you do with your body. No matter what may be going on, these areas are where you can always generate change.

You get to choose your perspective about what's happening. You get to choose whether life is happening *for* you or *against* you. You get to choose whether you double down on closure or allow the breath to slow and deepen if only slightly.

Even when you get triggered, and the tension and reactivity of fight-flight-freeze patterns get ignited, you always, in each moment, have the ability to come back into opening, connection, and allowing. Soften your body and let your breath come more fluidly. The more you practice, the more this becomes automatic. Then, instead of subconsciously going into closure and shutting yourself off from your Life Force, you witness those moments and can make a new choice. Soften the body and stay open. Let the experience of this moment in, even if it feels scary or painful. Inhale beyond the fear and the pain, and exhale the tension so the emotions can move.

We are not here to do life perfectly. We are here to choose again and again, to be love in our most difficult moments. Be patient with yourself. Your brain can change.

You can practice this new consciousness by doing the first part of a 3-Step Process for Instant Healing, which I call the *Instant Elevation* technique. The first of the three steps is Awareness.

Daily Integration Exercise 1: The Drop In

- Drop into your body; feel sensation in your body.

- Bring your attention to your physical body; feel and sense what is happening.

- This can be as simple as saying: *Hi, body. Here we are. How are you?*

This focus of attention alone changes your brain function and your physiology. When your awareness is only outside you, paying attention to the threats or the circumstances you are trying to change, the fear physiology is ignited. When you bring your attention back into your body, even partially, it ignites the relaxation response and ignites self-healing.

This is a new conversation you have within your own system. It opens the lines of communication between you and your body. It brings your awareness to a new level of tuning in. In the final chapter of this book, we get into a deeper experience of using Instant Elevation to ignite even deeper healing. Until then, practice this simple step so you develop deeper awareness.

Set your alarm for three to five times a day as you read this book to check in with your body. It could be a three-second check-in. It could be a three-minute check-in. Just do the practice regularly—however it's easiest for you to establish a routine.

Your neural pathways change when you develop this new habit and practice it day after day. New neural pathways develop within weeks of this type of practice. This sets up the circuitry that brings awareness of what is going on in your body. After you have taken on this practice, when you get triggered, you'll notice more readily whether you are in shutdown and closure or tension. You'll have more compassion for yourself in that moment.

Compassion greatly assists the healing process because it brings you back into openness and connection with Source Intelligence and out of that closure that starves you. You now are aware of a choice in each moment — whether you remain open to the flow of Source Intelligence and healing or you remain in closure and see what that choice will ultimately create. You do not have to open. You get to choose. It's not wrong to close. It generates circumstances that help clarify what results from your choices.

Your experience is for your awakening. It's all happening so you begin to see.

You can stay in closure as long as you choose to. The good news is life is going to keep waking you up—sometimes by kicking you in the butt—because what closure ultimately creates is more hardship, more chaos, more problems, more fear and, ultimately, more disease, pain, and symptoms.

Your body is on board for your awakening process, and that's why it is getting your attention. Your body reflects your closure through illness, pain, and stuck situations. It's like a movie screen carrying the projection of what's going on within you. What shows up as lack or scarcity—not having enough time, energy, or money—is a reflection of something being held in your energy system. These circumstances are simply reflecting a choice you're making—usually unconsciously—that you can now change. This is how your system is letting you see what you are, in fact, creating. If you do not recognize you are closing yourself off, if you suppress the awareness and allow closure to persist, your body speaks up, in a whisper or a scream if it has to, to show you it is time to open up again.

If you accept what I'm sharing here and you listen and tune in, things will change. When you see your symptoms as a reminder to soften and relax, you are going to allow yourself to open back to Source Intelligence and allow healing to happen.

This was a big part of my healing process. During the autoimmune illness I had in medical school, I had severe back pain. Every time I would feel that back pain, I would immediately think: *Oh no! I am in trouble. It is getting worse, I will never make it, I am never going to heal, it will not be okay. After everything I have done, it's still there.*

I felt powerless and hopeless every time I felt back pain. I began to realize that I could do the opposite. Every time I felt the severe pain and spasm in my back, I told my body: *Hi body, I am right here. It is okay to feel this, you can relax, it is okay to let go. I love you. I fully accept myself; it is okay to feel what I feel right now.*

My body would unwind, soften, and relax, and the pain dissolved until I no longer had any pain syndrome whatsoever.

Unconscious to Conscious:
Your Symptoms Can Awaken You

Everything in this book is an invitation to be in a new relationship with your body, your sensations, your physiology, and your health. Your body reflects what's going on within you. It shows you all the unconscious patterns, old traumas, resentments, hurts, and past experiences that are not resolved emotionally. It will show you specifically what you have been holding that you are ready to let go.

If you let this be an open communication and allow your body to talk to you, any unresolved issues move more swiftly.

If you keep making it wrong that you are having symptoms or if you are angry with your body for being in pain or letting you down or betraying you, then you are missing the whole point, and the body becomes more inflamed.

Your cells are listening. They reflect everything you are holding. Most of the stuff you are holding in your system is not conscious. Whether it was an argument you had last week with your mother, not having your needs met when you were three years old and were punished instead, or some severe trauma that left you feeling completely powerless, these memories are still stored in your body. They are not there to punish you but to serve as a placeholder. You can go back and resolve them, make a new choice, and find the strength and compassion you did not have when they occurred.

Resolving and releasing stored emotions can be easy. Emotions are energy-in-motion. They are meant to move through your system within twelve to fifteen seconds. They can enrich your life. However, some people hold on to emotions for decades and suffer the consequences. When you feel and sense your body with this awareness practice, checking in, physically softening the shoulders and belly, letting the breath flow more fluidly and say: *Hi, body* a few times a day, you feel and sense a lot of things that you may have blocked.

Find a special bonus of an audio file of this practice at DrKimD.com/BYOHbonuses, just for readers of this book.

You may feel fear that was previously a background worry. You may experience shame that was previously a low level of inadequacy. You may feel despair because you have lost a loved one or feel alone. You may have developed an addiction to work or to social media to keep you distracted from those feelings. I am inviting you to drop into the body, connect with the sensations, and breathe those feelings instead of suppressing them. The body will breathe the energy out.

As an electromagnetic being, those energies make up your system. You may overwork, distract, or take up an addiction as a way to suppress your feelings, but they are still actively creating limitation and illness in your life. The path to wholeness, true freedom, and vitality is to allow those energies to move. This may mean meeting that space of despair, fear, and loneliness. This process is not meant to have you re-live the past, but a way to have compassion for that part of you who still resides there now. Your energy body is a conglomerate of unconscious memories and things you have learned. You may have learned: *I am not worthy unless I achieve. I do not matter unless I work hard. I should do for others and ignore myself.*

When you drop in and practice awareness, you become aware of the patterns and programs at play in your life. This may be uncomfortable or overwhelming, but if you remember the purpose of awareness is to allow a clearing, you are more willing to lean into the patterns and programs and breathe, and that clears the way for the energy to move. A lot of the activity in your system stems from unconscious programs you can access right now, even though they may have happened decades ago. You do not need to identify your illness to access all the emotions right here, right now. The body only lives in the now. The body shows you where the emotions are.

When you drop in and become aware, you sense and feel what is here in the now. Meet this experience with compassion because this is what harmonizes those densities, those lower-frequency energies, and allows them to release.

We are made of pure energy, and it behooves us to understand how energy functions and how our energy body works. We may spend years trying to understand and change the physical world. We try to change our bodies by putting a ton of energy into dieting or treatments only to realize those efforts are limited to the physical level. If you put even a little bit of effort into learning how energy works and how your energy body functions, you will have a much bigger payoff.

In the physical world, the accepted ways to maintain good health keep changing. What you were supposed to eat five years ago is not at all what you are supposed to eat today. And so, we get confused. The world of the energy body is very simple, very fluid, very easy to learn, and it has an exponentially bigger payoff.

Three Functions of Your Energy Body

The energy body has three distinct functions:

- First, you are a *receptor*. You are constantly receiving and registering information and Intelligence from your environment.

- Second, you are a *transmitter*. Your body is emitting an electromagnetic field that has an impact on the world around you and sends a communication.

- Third, you are a *transmuter*. Your body can change and shift or transmute energy back to its highest and purest form.

As an energy receptor, what you focus on expands. Your body receives billions of bits of information every moment about the outside world, what is happening within your body, and even what is going on with your family, no matter where they are.

Most people do not let in all of this information. People are only letting in information matching their concept that they are a physical, separate being. They have been taught they can only know what they learn from a book or from what is happening in their immediate environment. They block all other information.

But what if you could get information about anything you want just by asking and *tuning in?*

You can experiment with receiving information by asking:

How is my child or family member doing right now?

Will this supplement bring health to my body?

or

Which action can I take now to increase the revenue in my business?

And you can receive the answers to those questions.

When I first learned about this receptivity, I was an osteopathic medical student in my second year. I was working with my partner Jen while we were being tested on our ability to do osteopathic manipulation of the spine. We had to evaluate our partner's body and diagnose the position of the spine, and then say what we would do to bring it back into a neutral alignment. I ran my hands up and down Jen's back several times, concentrating on one area of her back, thinking: *Oh God, I have no idea what is going on here.*

After a few times of doing this, I said to the tester, "I do not know what she has going on, but let's say, for example, that her fifth thoracic segment was sidebent right and rotated right."

The tester, Dr. Gretchen Sibley, an amazing osteopath in Maine, promptly put her notepad down, got up, and walked over to where we were working. She put her hands on Jen's back and said to me in a frustrated tone, "Kim, you ran your hands up and down Jen's back three times, and your hands went up to this exact segment where the lesion is. Then you said, 'Well I don't know,' but then you called out the exact lesion of what is going on in her spine."

In that moment, I was awestruck that my system was receiving all kinds of information, but I was blocking it because I did not believe I could know it. I had unconsciously registered exactly what was going on in Jen's body. Although my hands went there, I discounted it and did not let myself register it consciously. That moment changed everything in my life. I immediately, then and there, decided I was going to let information in, even if it did not make sense according to the construct of reality I had been taught—the one that said I am a physical, solid, separate being, and I cannot know this.

I have grown in my abilities exponentially since then. Now, I allow myself to be aware of conditions within my patient's body on the other side of the world. By tuning in, I can be aware of the root cause of my community member's tinnitus—ringing in the ears—even though I have never met her and only seen a few lines of what she wrote in a social media post.

As a receptor, you have the ability to tune the dial to the specific kind of information you want to receive. That dial you are tuning is your focus of attention.

I use this ability to ask what would make the most difference for my patient.

For instance:

What does my patient need to hear?

What is the root cause of this problem?

What would make the biggest difference for her healing?

I can immediately let myself have that awareness. It doesn't come to me in a full sentence, but unconsciously I will register a feeling, sensation, piece of information, or a question that helps us immediately get to the root cause. We can tune that dial by focusing our awareness. When you ask a question, you let in a specific kind of information that matches that question.

Another way to focus your awareness is to concentrate on the area where you feel a pain or symptom. Instead of responding with the fear, focus on the area with the thoughts: *I love you. It is okay to feel exactly what you are feeling right now.* Because you are focusing on a different kind of presence, you are letting new information come into that area of your body, and that alone can resolve the tension, pain, and illness.

Receptor is the first function of your energy body, and you can start to gently play with it by letting yourself be a better receiver. Focus your attention on what you want to achieve or feel, rather than what is wrong. Let go of focusing on what you *do not* want and shift your focus onto what you *do* want. Your receptive energy body will bring you that awareness.

The second function of your energy body is to be a *Transmitter*. The HeartMath Institute has a wealth of information about transmission. Your electromagnetic energy body creates an electromagnetic field and sends a signal to your cells, your body, and your environment. That energy can be measured up to ten feet away from the body and calibrates with your emotional state. If we are in joy, love, acceptance, and well-being, maybe thinking about someone or something we love, we emit a higher electromagnetic frequency. If we are frustrated, feeling angry, or hopeless, we emit a lower electromagnetic transmission. We have the ability to detect this and correlate it with emotions. This electromagnetic signal is felt by your cells, where it creates an immediate chemical physiologic shift and even impacts your DNA—your genetic code—and your genetic functioning. It is also transmitted outward and impacts people around you. They have a feeling of ease, well-being, or warmth when they are in your presence.

The opposite is also true. If you think: *My husband is so difficult*, he is going to have a feeling of protection, and he is going to go into even more closure and a narcissistic pattern.

When you start paying attention to your electromagnetic field and understand that you are a transmitter, you realize you have a much greater leverage point to impact your circumstances and your body. You impact everything around you, and your world will serve as the reflection of the signals you are putting out.

You can choose what you emit, and transmit more of the pure love that you are. Then you allow that presence more fully in the reflection in the world. You can bring out the best in others. You can allow a higher manifestation of opportunities and abundance. If you don't like what you see in your life, remember a large part of what you see is due to your own transmission, and you can change this.

The third function of your energy body is that of a *Transmuter*. We go into more detail on this later, but basically energy vibrates at a certain frequency that can be shifted. Through your interaction with it, energy can be moved into a higher frequency.

All energy wants to move. That's its nature. Life is in constant motion and change. How you interact with life will determine how life is. What you resist persists. It's not the lower negative emotions that have a detrimental effect on your health; it is your resistance to feeling those emotions and letting them move through you. When you allow transmutation, you are coming into a more harmonious relationship with that energy.

It may seem to you like there is no way you could let in and be at peace with shame, fear, despair, or depression. You think you have to fight it. You have to block out. You have to resist it. But remember all energy wants to move. Emotion is energy in motion. When you allow energy to flow, it becomes a heightened emotion. What you resist becomes destructive. It feels like a negative emotion. If you embrace your despair, your fear, or your worry, instead of trying to make those emotions go away, your body will let the energy move through, and you will feel lighter.

Think about a challenge coming up in your life—the biggest one getting your attention right now. Is it a person, or your body, or work, or money? Bring that into your awareness.

Breathe to welcome in the sensations you are feeling right now. Do you feel tension in your chest? Do you feel pressure in your head? Do you feel a rush of anxiety?

Whatever you feel, it is okay, but choose to feel it, to welcome it. Breathe more fully into it and let it expand.

When you do a practice like this, the energy moves and resolves. Because you release the resistance, the energy can move, and that emotion dissolves.

You will find more practice with this in the audios included with this book at DrKimD.com/BYOHbonuses

Transmutation is one of the most powerful tools I use to assist people to resolve disease, illness, anxiety, depression, fatigue, and pain because we are working with the deepest energies keeping those things in place. When you remember your body is a transmuter, and that is how you are designed to function, you can let yourself use the functionality a lot more freely.

Your Three Nervous Systems

We tend to think of our nervous system as one network that sends signals throughout the body—the brain is connecting to the body to tell it what to do. In the Western medical model, we have awareness of two parts of the nervous system—*voluntary* and *involuntary*.

In the voluntary system, when you want to reach for a glass of water and drink it, your brain is telling your hand to reach for the glass, grasp it, and bring it to your mouth. Your brain knows exactly what to do because you are making a conscious choice to tell your hand what to do.

The involuntary nervous system controls your heart rate and the tone or pressure in your vessels so your blood pressure stays at the right level. The involuntary nervous system controls your metabolism and digestion, making urine and detoxifying.

The involuntary autonomic nervous system is made of the sympathetic and the parasympathetic components. Both of these are involuntary functions of your nervous system or autonomic nervous system. *Autonomic is automatic.* I do not have to think about it; it is not under conscious control.

The third part of the nervous system is the *meridian network*. It is not appreciated by the Western medical system, but it is extremely important in Eastern medicine. If you have ever had acupuncture or acupressure, you are aware of the great power of clearing the meridian channels to improve their functions. This is the part of the nervous system I am going to talk about more because it is where we are able to gather a vast amount of information about what is happening in the body. Your electromagnetic state or electromagnetic frequency can be detected through this third nervous system. The meridian channels are either open, sending a strong signal to your body, muscles, and organs, allowing healthy functions—or they can be closed, showing disease and lack of health in different areas of the body.

When you want to get a sense of what is happening electromagnetically, you can use this nervous system to get information from the body to guide what you are doing.

The third nervous system is a more subtle nervous system—one that governs powerfully over everything happening in the body. These have been known for many years; however, in a 2019 issue of the *Evidence-Based Complementary and Alternative Medicine* journal, Norbet Maurer, et al. published anatomical dissections demonstrating these pathways in the physical body (Maurer et al. 2019). The meridians are energy pathways well documented and well understood in the Eastern medicine model.

Kinesiology: Tuning Into Your Body Senses for Awareness

One of the ways you can develop more awareness of what is going on in the body is through the practice of kinesiology. It is commonly used in Eastern medicine and is becoming more commonly used in Western medicine by many chiropractors and other practitioners.

Kinesiology is a way of getting information from the body at a level beyond the conscious mind. A person may not consciously know their liver meridian is blocked, but the body definitely knows, and you will see a weakening of certain muscles and a strengthening of certain other muscles when this occurs.

Kinesiology allows us to obtain information by observing whether the body goes strong or weak in response to certain stimuli. This is referred to as *muscle testing*. If a person holds out their arm while the tester attempts to push it down, it may strongly resist the pressure and remain outstretched, or it may weaken and fall to the person's side.

The body's energy field, and therefore physical strength, will be strengthened with the truth, such as the person saying, "My name is _____" and saying their correct name. It will be weakened with a lie, such as saying, "My name is Mickey Mouse."

This insight can be very useful as a way to tune into information otherwise too subtle or unknown to us. We can ask the body's Intelligence about what's underlying an illness or an issue and get a sense of where to work, what would be beneficial, or what needs to be removed. The response is not governed consciously by the subject; even if they exert effort, they will not be able to resist the pressure of the one doing the testing unless that is the authentic response from the body-mind.

Most people have not developed the sensitivity to tune into information at this level; however, highly attuned practitioners are able to receive this information without necessarily going through the kinesiologic process. I do not personally use kinesiology in my practice. I've learned to directly let the information and insight into my awareness. This is a skill most people can develop. It took years of study, focus, and intention to develop this, but it is a true gift I use every day and has served me and my clients immensely.

Kinesiology studies the body's ability to register and respond to the energy of what is around it. For example, a person may have no conscious awareness of whether a particular medication or supplement will be helpful or harmful for them, but the wisdom in their body knows. If you hold that medicine or supplement up to your solar plexus and ask, "Will this be beneficial for me?" then we muscle test, the body will respond with a yes or a no. It will go weak or strong to give us the awareness.

Strong means yes: You hold up your arm, and it resists downward pressure. The arm stays up. If we hold a substance that would be beneficial and supportive to the body, we see the body become strong when we do strength testing. The body's electromagnetic field senses the quality and impact of that substance. It is already registering the positive effects of that item. The person might not even know what is in that glass or in the pill, but the innate Intelligence of the body absolutely knows. It is letting in the electromagnetic energy of the substance and detecting its effects.

Weak means no: With just a little bit of pressure on the arm, it goes down. You can't hold it up. Even if you tell yourself you're not going to let it be pushed, and you brace yourself against the pressure, the tester easily sends your arm down. The weakness only lasts for a second. It does not impact the voluntary nervous system. It's impacting the electromagnetics, which have a more subtle effect.

The body's Intelligence can register the information even when it's kept covered inside an envelope and there is no way the person could possibly be consciously aware of what is inside. This third part of the nervous system is constantly communicating with us and can register information and Intelligence that can be very helpful in uncovering the root causes of diseases and making wise treatment choices.

There are many ways this type of testing can be used. We can use this to examine the impact of our intelligence, thoughts, and beliefs. You can instruct someone to hold their arm out and have them say, "I love myself and I can do anything." If the person stays strong, the electromagnetics are strengthening the neural pathways and the meridian channels. It is feeding the nervous system with Life Force, and muscles stay strong.

If you have that same person say, "I am a loser and I will never make it," their system will immediately go weak and the muscle test will demonstrate this.

Try it right now with a friend. It's important to be well-hydrated. There are other factors also affecting this testing, but we're going to keep it very simple and basic here. You can find a video demonstration of this in the book resources.

Go to DrKimD.com/BYOHbonuses to view the video and witness the kinesiology process.

It is encouraging to directly witness how our thoughts, beliefs, and words immediately affect our bodies. This process demonstrates that the innate Intelligence of our body knows what is beneficial to us and what is not.

You do not need to do a kinesiologic test to get this information. Maybe you start with this physical practice to let your system become more adept with this kind of communication. It can be very strange and mind-blowing to many simply realizing there is innate wisdom in the body. Let yourself become adept with letting in information through new pathways. Then we can begin letting the information in more directly, where it pops directly into your awareness with clarity and certainty. I do this all the time.

We can tune into our intuition, and we may sense a *Ding! Ding! Ding! Yes, I am going to take that supplement,* or *I am going call that person,* or *it is time for me to stop this medication,* because the Intelligence of the body can send you that signal and have you register that awareness. Kinesiology demonstrates there is innate Intelligence in your body. You can directly communicate with it, with yes or no questions for all kinds of information about your health, your choices, and your life. You just have to become more receptive. Listen deeply. Softening the body and slowing the breath are essential for this. Keep practicing Drop In, the first Daily Integration exercise from page **91** in this book. Begin asking questions and letting the information in. We'll add to that exercise to deepen your receptivity.

Don't try to answer the question. Just ask the question and tune into the frequency of the question.

Kinesiologic testing also demonstrates that your thoughts immediately and significantly impact the physiological functioning of your body. When you embody truths—*I am powerful, life is on my side, life is happening on my behalf, it is okay for me to trust and let go*—you routinely find your body is strong. You may even feel an immediate lightness when you hold these thoughts.

You can start playing with those affirmations, talking to your cells and letting your body know *it is okay to feel what you feel. I fully love and accept you.* You will ignite harmonization and power in your body right now. All three parts of your nervous system are affected by your thoughts, beliefs, and substances in and around you. They are also affected by suppressed emotions you may not be aware of.

The third nervous system is the most subtly affected and subtly communicative; it gives more direct insight into the messages from the innate Intelligence of the body. When we neglect this, as has been done in Western medicine, we lose a deeper communication with the body and can feel like we're in a never-ending no man's land when trying to understand an illness.

Not for you anymore. Whenever you feel you are in a conundrum, caught between a rock and a hard place, dealing with an unsolvable problem, soften. Don't buy into it.

- Get curious.

- Ask a question.

- Receive.

CHAPTER THREE

Don't Believe What You Think

Let's go deeper. Let's keep changing our perspective so we change our reality. You are deepening into the technology of your body. To be your own healer, you must release everything you think you are and everything you think is true about everything. You must begin to see from truth instead of from programming.

Often, we do not realize what we think of as reality is really just our perception. We aren't aware that many of the beliefs we hold—consciously or unconsciously—color the way we see and experience everything. Even the emotions we feel are a direct result of our own perception, not necessarily what's actually happening. We think what we see is true, but it's a conglomerate of all the programs, training, experiences, assumptions, and societal messaging that happen to us throughout our lives. Within ourselves, there is a part with a deeper knowing that goes far beyond everything we think, everything we have learned, and everything we believe. The thinking mind, made up of our personal beliefs, identities, memories, and experiences, is not the same as the knowing mind, which is where we find the True-Self.

Even as I write this book, I am prompted to move from the thinking mind into the knowing mind. I remember to soften my body so I enter this deeper space. This is the part of the mind that is the most powerful. It allows what's shared here to be from Universal Source Consciousness instead of Kim consciousness, which is far more limited. If we live only from the thinking mind, filled with our beliefs, thoughts, experiences, memories, perception, and training, we may completely miss out on our knowing mind and the awareness of what is a greater truth.

The current conventional medical and scientific models teach the body is a solid, separate, purely physical thing. We have a lot of ideas about how it responds, how it reacts, what it can do, and what it cannot do. We do not allow ourselves to appreciate it is a living thing, pure energy constantly changing, always in flux, and responding to everything around us. The body responds to the energy within us—specifically our own consciousness, thoughts, beliefs, and memories. The beliefs are like playlists in the background, always giving signals and commands that orchestrate how those cells behave and carry messages to every cell in our body. Are they in health and harmony, or are they in discord and disharmony, which leads to disease?

Everything depends on where your attention is placed.

You may not realize your dynamic, ever-changing and ever-receptive body has a lot more possibility and potential than what you believe or what the conventional medical perspective says. Recognize that your cells are listening—meaning they are being affected by the cellular environment, hormones, neural chemicals, and electromagnetic signals being sent—and this impacts how they function. When you see the body as pure energy, listening, responsive, and receptive, you realize you have a powerful leverage point with which to impact what is happening in your body, to impact what is happening cellularly, and to impact what is happening medically.

Look at these influences of your thoughts, beliefs, chemistry, emotions and all those signals going on throughout your body. These are powerful messages. *This is not a subtle effect; this is the prime determining factor that will dictate whether you exhibit health or disease.*

Psychoneuroimmunology: It's All Connected

Before I went to medical school, I attended an event called the Yankee Dental Congress. I went with my father, a prominent oral surgeon. This was a huge annual dental conference that took place in Boston where I grew up. My dad was a speaker at that event. I went to hear his talk, and we also attended some of the other presentations.

I attended a talk by Joan Borysenko, Ph.D. She spoke about MindBody Medicine—how our thoughts affect cells, how our beliefs send chemical signals that affect everything happening within our body, and how our body is a constantly changing receptor responding to all these energies. I will never forget what she said; it changed the whole course of my life.

I was completely and utterly fascinated with how she was putting together the scientific understanding of how everything is consciousness and is all connected—that things are not separate.

When I was in medical school, we studied the mind and the body separately. We studied the nervous system, the gastrointestinal system, the cardiac system, and so on. Your liver is over here doing its thing. Your brain is over there doing its thing. We never studied how they interact with each other. But in this science of *psycho-neuro-immun-ology* (psycho = thoughts and beliefs, neuro = brain and nervous system, immun = immune system, ology = study of) we understand thoughts and beliefs directly affect the brain and nervous system. They directly affect your immune system and whether you adequately fight off disease and stay healthy.

The immune system plays a direct role in keeping you free from pathogens and clearing infectious diseases. It is the system involved with the development of or resistance to cancer. All the systems are directly interrelated, meaning the chemical messengers from one system are not in any way separate from the other systems; they are the same messengers involved in all the different areas. The endocrine system is mixed in with this as well, so the study has come to be called *psycho-neuro-immuno-endocrinology*; however, the original name *psychoneuroimmunology* is typically still used for brevity.

The truth is all systems of the body are completely interrelated, intercommunicating, and directly connecting with each other. The science of psychoneuroimmunology shows these are not separate systems at all. Your thought directly affects your hormones and reproductive organs, determining whether you can become pregnant easily. Your beliefs and emotions directly affect the function of your immune system, which is directly related to your gut and your ability to absorb nutrients and stay healthy, resilient, and vibrant. The beliefs you hold can also determine whether you develop a bowel disease, if your bowels are inflamed and have intolerance to certain foods, or if you develop Crohn's disease or ulcerative colitis—serious diseases.

Your cells are fed either by the false matrix with its limited belief systems, or by the Infinite Self. Are you present to this Infinite Self—the expansive space of wonder and awe? Or are you functioning with only the small-self identity, who has no clue what the heck I'm talking about here?

All the things we are doing in medicine to fight disease and treat the symptoms are a drop in the bucket compared to the power in the interconnected communication system that so powerfully and immediately impacts the health of every cell. The entire system directly involves your beliefs and your emotions.

I was fascinated when I first learned this. Having already been an intuitive and empathic person, this all seemed to exactly match my own inner knowing about how the body worked. It was as if science was now validating everything I had already become aware of, and I became deeply impassioned by this work.

I bought every book on Dr. Borysenko's recommended reading list, and I studied everything I could. A year later at that same conference, her session filled the grand ballroom. There was standing room only because so many practitioners were eager to hear her speak. I had the awareness that many did not fully understand what this topic was really about. Even without that understanding, somewhere in our collective knowing we are intrigued because we know intrinsically that this is the Truth. We are awakening.

We may be shown a limited view of the body with its separate, solid systems, but deep down we know there is a more powerful leverage point to understand the orchestration of the body and have an impact on it to influence health. Somewhere deep inside, we yearn to emerge into that way of practicing medicine. I was profoundly inspired and knew my future in some way would lie in the field of MindBody Medicine.

Years later in medical school, I developed a severe autoimmune disease. I had severe joint pain, fatigue, lethargy, headaches, and brain fog and felt aches and chills intermittently, as if I were in the early stage of getting the flu. Over the course of about a year, I went to every doctor I could possibly go to, trying to find out what was wrong with me.

Eventually my labs showed some abnormalities, but no one could understand how to fix my problem or even identify it. I kept getting worse and worse. I kept revisiting this idea of MindBody Medicine. I understood on some level my thoughts and my emotions were involved in the process, but I could not get a handle on how to change that. I had read all the books on how the body heals itself and how the mind and body are connected, but I did not have a good how-to guide to leverage this and make changes so my body could heal.

Ultimately, that was the inspiration for my first book, the *MindBody Toolkit*, which describes ten tools to use anywhere, anytime, to immediately shift your body toward a state of greater health. I knew there was a lot of research and science about this, but what I didn't know was what to do with it. When I wrote my first book, it was about specific things you could do at any moment to leverage this power. That information would have benefitted me, and I knew it was a major piece missing from the puzzle of self-healing.

I was at my wit's end trying to apply this understanding and struggled with figuring my way through it. *The mind and body are connected; the body can heal itself—but how do I activate this in my body?* I knew the obscure illness nobody could name was somehow created from what was happening within me, in my unconscious, but I had no way to directly change it. It took well over a year to finally get a specific diagnosis.

I was sent to an allergist who had been recommended by the infectious disease specialist, who then injected every kind of known allergen into my skin, only to find I reacted against almost all of them. He came up with the whole diagnosis and proposed solution. "Here you go!" he said, "You have a rare, obscure form of late-onset Juvenile Rheumatoid Arthritis."

I was devastated. It sounded like a death sentence. I would have to make serious lifestyle changes. I would not run again. I would have to control my living environment. No curtains, no rugs. There would be lots of cleaning with special solutions. My head was spinning.

I thought I would dissolve into a puddle of despair. I was a medical student about to begin hospital rotations with no control over my living environment in the hospital living quarters. The life I had imagined was falling apart. How was I going to carry on living my dream if I was not able to move through the world without getting terribly sick?

This moment was short-lived, however. After that initial wave of despair, I thought: *Wait a minute—what if what he's saying is not true for me?* This immediately brought a sense of lightness because I knew his perspective and the context he was functioning within were indeed limited and not true for me. I knew better. I knew my body was not a static thing and a disease state was not something happening to me I had to protect myself from, but rather *my body was responding to something.*

I had never had an allergy to any of these environmental factors before. I had gone through most of my life not allergic to anything. All of a sudden, I was inflamed against all these particular things where I had not been inflamed before?

I asked myself: *What would it take for me to resolve this? What would it take for my body to go back to the state of living in total harmony with all these environmental factors?* That is when I opened to possibility. Something shifted. I no longer felt like collapsing into a puddle on the floor. I felt a lightness.

I thanked the doctor for his input and went on my own merry way. I never took any prescribed medications. I never made any proposed lifestyle changes. I decided I was going to have a different conversation with my body. I realized my body was not my enemy. It was trying to show me something. It was inflamed, and there was a reason. I could trust my body instead of fighting it. I would ask and listen. I would soften and receive.

That very day I took a long walk on the beach and began asking: *Body, what is going on? What do I need to know? What is right about this that I am not getting?*

I had finally stopped asking: *What is wrong with me? What is wrong with me? What is wrong with me?* which had only generated an even more intense stress state. Instead, I started asking: *What is right about this that I am not getting?* I could feel myself dropping into my body more in partnership to stay curious and receive what my body was trying to show me. If my MindBody system was created from wisdom, then I could let that wisdom come in, but I could not do it from the tension of trying to dig and dig for the answers. I would have to surrender. I had to soften and finally be receptive to this body I had been fighting against and so afraid of.

Thoughts Are Things: Chemical Messengers and Electromagnetic Frequencies

I learned from Dr. Joan Borysenko and psychoneuroimmunology that thoughts are things. They are chemical signals that affect our cells. Whether hormones, inflammatory markers, or neurochemicals, the chemical messengers from each system cross over into all the other systems and are either going to enhance or decrease the health of those cells and those systems.

Beyond the chemical, which is a physical messaging system, the *molecules of emotion* carry the frequency of our thoughts and have electromagnetic properties. When we think of a nerve impulse traveling down the nerve to the synapse, it sends a signal to another nerve cell, having an end effect.

Now I'm going to get a little nerdy and science-y. I've been warned by some, including my own mother, *not to talk about the atoms and particles stuff because it's too weird and you'll lose your audience; just talk about the physical stuff and keep it normal.*

That works for some; however, I have found such deep truths lie in the subtle energies, it's worth it to *weird out* a bit and go deeper into what science has demonstrated about our inner power. Hang with me here; I'll do my best to make this very applicable to you and your desire for self-healing.

Unlike chemical messengers that travel in physical space and time, electromagnetic signals behave differently. What we have seen clinically is that the body will *instantaneously* register information on the energetic level. This means rather than a signal being sent, traveling through space and time to get to its destination, and then having impact, electromagnetic signals are *instantaneous*.

When we think of those three parts of your nervous system we talked about earlier: the voluntary nervous system, the involuntary nervous system (parasympathetic and sympathetic), and then the electromagnetic nervous system, this third system registers and transmits information in a very different way.

At the electromagnetic level, all energy is connected. There is no separation between one molecule and another. There is a seamless *cohesion* between parts of one atom and another. The smallest parts that make up the atoms—electrons, photons, neutrons—are constantly moving around, shared between the atoms. They're not separate.

In experiments [1]by Dr. Nicholas Gesin at the University of Geneva in 1997, a photon—a unit of light—was split in

1 *Salart, D.; Baas, A.; Branciard, C.; Gisin, N; Zbinden, H. (2008). "Testing the speed of 'spooky action at a distance'". Nature. **454** (7206): 861–864. arXiv:0808.3316. doi:10.1038/ nature07121. PMID 18704081. S2CID 4401216.*

two, and the two photons were sent seven miles in either direction. Scientists saw that whatever they did to one photon *instantaneously* showed up in the activity of the other photon—even though they were fourteen miles apart. There is no way these units of energy could have communicated with each other through space so quickly. The energy of one part is *connected* to all other parts and, therefore, can instantaneously transmit the new frequency. This connection between the apparently separated particles is called *quantum entanglement*. It indicates the particles remain somehow connected no matter how physically separate they appear to be.

You are the same. Your thoughts are carriers of energy and consciousness. They are chemical signals as I've outlined above, but they also carry *frequency*. They carry a transmission of information. Different kinds of thoughts have different

- Tittel, W.; Brendel, J.; Gisin, N.; Zbinden, H. (1999). "Long-distance Bell-type tests using energy-time entangled photons". Phys. Rev. A. **59** (6): 4150–4163. arXiv:quant-ph/9809025. doi:10.1103/PhysRevA.59.4150. S2CID 119095575.

- Gisin, N.; Zbinden, H. (1999). "Bell inequality and the locality loophole: Active versus passive switches". Phys. Lett. A. **264** (2–3): 103–107. arXiv:quant-ph/9906049. doi:10.1016/S0375-9601(99)00807-5. S2CID 15383228.

- Zbinden, H.; Brendel, J.; Gisin, N.; Tittel, W. (2001). "Experimental test of nonlocal quantum correlation in relativistic configurations" (PDF). Physical Review A. **63** (2): 022111. arXiv:quant-ph/0007009. doi:10.1103/PhysRevA.63.022111. S2CID 44611890.

- Stefanov, A.; Zbinden, H.; Gisin, N.; Suarez, A. (2002). "Quantum correlations with spacelike separated beam splitters in motion: Experimental test of multisimultaneity". Phys. Rev. Lett. **88** (12): 120404. arXiv:quant-ph/0110117. doi:10.1103/PhysRevLett.88.120404. PMID 11909434. S2CID 119522191.

rates of vibration and resonance. For example, if we construct thoughts like: *I love myself fully; I accept myself completely; it is okay for me to be free in the world*—these have a high-vibrational frequency and a positive, strengthening effect on the body and nervous system.

The HeartMath Institute has shown our emotions in fact impact our DNA in ways that can enhance or limit our health. According to a study done in 1994 by Drs. Glen Rein and Rollin McCraty, higher emotional states like love and joy were shown to have an opening effect, unwinding our DNA, which enhances our immune function, DHEA production and hormone balance, and overall health. Lower emotions such as anger, fear, frustration, or shame, were shown to have a compacting effect on our DNA, winding it more tightly (Rein and McCraty 1994). This was shown to have a suppressive impact on immune function, DHEA levels and hormone balance, and overall health. Our emotions have been shown to impact the state of our DNA directly and significantly. Emotion changes matter. This is the power within the technology of your body.

All thoughts have a certain vibration, a certain electromagnetic frequency. If we have thoughts like: *Oh my God, what is wrong with me?! Nothing I am doing is working. I am trying to see more and more doctors, but nobody has any answers for me,* this transmits a different vibrational frequency that has a suppressive effect on our system. Beyond the chemical messengers of our thoughts and emotions, these electromagnetic frequencies are seen to be even more powerful—even more immediate and instantaneously transmitted. And importantly, they transmit a signal that goes beyond the body. They are not limited to the space we see as the physical structure of the body. In fact, we can measure these electromagnetic frequencies up to eight to ten feet away from the body and get a read on whether someone is in a state of joy, relaxation, or peace. We can also read if someone is in a lower frequency state like anger, fear, or embarrassment.

Changing Your Frequency Changes Your Cells, DNA, and Transmission

Your electromagnetic field has a direct impact on what is happening in your cells. Specific cellular changes occur depending on your vibrational frequency. If you walk around most of your life living in joy and peace, you are in acceptance. You are receiving life as it goes. There is flow. That electromagnetic vibration activates health, enhances detoxification and removal of waste products, and stimulates the robust function of your cells and organs and the overall health of your body.

The opposite is also true. If you hold yourself in fear, constantly trying to make things work, overwhelmed but trying to do more, unwilling to let go because you are so scared; or angry, constantly blaming everyone else for your plight, you are in resistance. Your cellular and organ function is dampened and eventually develops disease.

It is fascinating, though, that the electromagnetic field affects even your DNA. Conventional medicine has viewed genes as a static situation. Most have held the perspective if you have genes for a particular disease, you are probably going to get that disease. The truth is, what is even more powerful than the genes themselves is the *environment* that activates or deactivates those genes. The study of *epigenetics* examines the science that governs our gene expression—determining whether certain genes are turned on or turned off, whether the DNA is repaired easily, or is in disrepair and manifests in disease.

When we are habitually in higher frequencies, we are deactivating those genes known to cause cancer, diabetes, obesity, and depression. We are activating genes that help us stay resilient, repair the body, and help us heal. When we habitually hold lower frequencies, suppressing the lower emotions of shame, guilt, fear, or anger, this impacts our genes in a negative way. It will activate the genes for disease very directly and impair the body's ability to heal itself at the genetic level.

This impact is not only local, but also remote. We've seen in multiple studies how our *intention* impacts another person physically, mentally, and emotionally. When I first started studying MindBody Medicine, I was fascinated by this. I learned about the Byrd Prayer studies, which demonstrated the effects of nonlocal healing using focused intention. Cardiologist Randolph Byrd published a study in the *Southern Medical Journal* in 1988 called "Positive Therapeutic Effects of Intercessory Prayer in a Coronary Care Unit Population," which demonstrated patients admitted to the cardiac care unit who had no idea they were being prayed for had fewer symptoms and a shorter duration of stay than those who were not being prayed for. They physiologically measured the impact of the remote intentions being sent by a distant person who only had their name and diagnosis and would send healing intentions. This was one of the first well-done scientific studies clearly demonstrating remote healing and interconnection (Byrd 1988).

Many similar studies have been done since that time to successfully replicate these data, demonstrating the powerful effects of remote healing and the power of intention.

I remember sharing this information with some of my pre-med colleagues at Harvard University, where we were all taking courses. They looked at me like I had three heads. The other students scoffed at me and argued this was impossible. I was very surprised at the strong conclusions they held about what was or was not possible and how avidly they argued for their limiting perspectives rather than being open to considering new information. When I later pulled up the studies from the library and presented them, they were literally speechless. One apologized and was clearly moved to have witnessed his own foolishness. The others never spoke to me again.

I have since found many doctors who are, in fact, open to new ideas and perspectives and new ways of seeing. These practitioners have courage and are actively exploring what truly supports healing. I have also found some who are unable to do this for various reasons. I have always felt that my greatest responsibilities as a physician are to stay open, explore without prejudice, and question everything, so I can get closer to the truth of what will create the most healing. I've found an immense body of work to demonstrate the true power that we each have to heal.

The *observer effect* is the effect of your thoughts and intentions extending beyond your body. Your energy body carries this signal and radiates outward beyond your physical body and impacts physical matter. It has a direct impact on everyone and everything around you. The HeartMath Institute has demonstrated in *Science of the Heart: Exploring the Role of the Heart in Human Performance*[2] that a person projecting their positive or negative thoughts onto a monitored person in a separate room changes that other person's emotional state, chemical output, and brain activity. There were also changes in that second person's electromagnetic frequency. Additionally, they noted subjective changes where the monitored person felt a sense of joy or love when someone sent remote intentions for their well-being.

> *The very act of observation is an act of creation.*
> ~ Gregg Braden, *The Divine Matrix*

We do not live in a vacuum. We live in a space filled with energy. The frequency of the energy around us impacts our bodies. It's helpful to remember this because we can choose to impact others in a positive way when we remember they are also responding to *our* energy field. People readily acknowledge a dog will sense someone's fear and is more likely to attack someone emoting that fear. It's the same with people. When you harbor anger around others, they can feel you. When you carry low-frequency energies, others around you are more likely to behave negatively toward you.

What will you do with this information?

---

2 Volume 2. Published by the HeartMath Institute, 2016.

It's up to you. You are a creator. If you cultivate a state of joy and peace, accepting yourself fully, you are directly *electromagnetically* affecting the people around you, making it more likely they will be loving, kind, and generous. This happens even if they are not that way around anyone else.

Making this shift in your way of living and thinking is not about being positive; it's about doing your best to be a space of love and compassion for everything you think is negative.

Your vibrational field also determines the aspects of others you bring out. Have you ever had an experience with a crabby person, and someone else says, "Oh, she's so sweet," and you wonder if you are talking about the same person? That's because the person behaves differently in the other person's field than how they've behaved around you. A person expresses the best or worst in themselves, depending on the impact you have on them.

My husband uses this awareness all the time. He'll walk to our local post office—a place where people notoriously have challenges with the service—and make friends with everyone. He'll send positive loving thoughts to the people behind the counter before he even walks in. He'll decide he's going to have a great experience, and he'll let whatever happens be accepted and embraced. When he enters, he'll be friendly and loving and let them know how much he appreciates their service. They adore him. They smile and go out of their way to take care of him. Interactions take a fraction of the time for him because he harmonizes the relationship first. He has an experience few ever have in that same situation. When we understand we are an electromagnetic field and we emanate a transmission that equals the sum of our own thoughts and emotions, we see how to leverage the Universe. We create our own reality depending on what we hold within us.

YOUR ATTENTION IS YOUR CREATIVE POWER— DON'T LET IT BE HIJACKED

Now that we understand the creative power we have to impact our surroundings and the people and spaces around us, we realize the Universe appears differently depending on what we ourselves are transmitting. We understand how important and powerful our personal frequency is in creating our lives. However, most of what is going on within us is unconscious. Only about 5% of our thoughts and beliefs are in our conscious awareness. About 95% of our thoughts and beliefs, and therefore our energy transmission, are unconscious.

That is why I was so unsuccessful the whole year I was trying to heal myself. I had no idea how much my unconscious beliefs were creating my unwanted reality and no clue what those thoughts and beliefs were. I had to look deep within myself to see what was creating problem after problem, working against my intentions for health.

It could have taken years of conventional therapy to try to change my unconscious beliefs and programming. That's because these beliefs, memories, traumas, and unconscious behaviors become deeply embedded in the system. Many people spend years trying to change their unconscious patterns and make minimal, if any, real change. Our electromagnetic field *can* impact and change our entire system at the deepest levels, and it can allow a massive shift within our unconscious patterns—and we can shift our electromagnetic frequency very quickly.

How do we enact this powerful transformation?

We shift our electromagnetic frequency immediately depending on where we focus our full attention. This happens immediately depending on *where we put our attention.*

Even if we have lots of negative thoughts and dense emotions repressed in our overall vibrational frequency, if we shift our attention to a higher frequency our electromagnetic field will immediately shift. Your *attention* is the fulcrum for everything being created right now in your cellular transmission, chemistry, brain function, and electromagnetic field. Your attention is your creative power. It sets the stage for what's being transmitted in your thoughts, emotions, overall energy, and frequency.

Changing where you place your attention and what you focus on initiates major changes in your brain, chemistry, nerve signals, and all your physiology. Practicing this change generates new patterns that allow you to remain in this state without trying. That's why it can feel difficult at first to think new thoughts like: *It will all be okay.* Your outer world may be reflecting the old beliefs: *Life is hard,* or, *I always get the short end of the stick.* However, with practice, we see things a new way. New neural pathways are laid down, and it becomes evident all is well. Then it is far easier for thoughts and emotions to align with that sense. At first, it takes energy to generate that change, but once we do, it becomes effortless.

Again, the practice is not about being positive. Have you ever tried to feel good when you feel really, really bad? It makes you feel worse. What you want to do instead is to change the frequency so you can let go of resistance. You move from: *I feel so bad, I don't want to feel like this* to: *I feel so bad, and it's okay to feel exactly what I feel now.*

It's a subtle quantum shift, but a huge amount of inner opening.

One practice I've learned that has greatly helped me do this is Ether Hicks's Focus Wheel process. Rather than trying to "be positive" and grab on to thoughts you clearly think are crap, you go slightly higher, reaching for a slightly higher thought, a slightly higher frequency, one you can percolate with and let in from exactly where you are. Instead of telling yourself a bunch of "positive" thoughts your system will bump out as junk—which I think of as putting ice cream on top of poop!—you appreciate where you are and reach for something you *can* embrace.

This works great when you're feeling low. For example, if I'm feeling miserable and hopeless, thinking low thoughts like: *It will never work out*, it would be unkind to tell myself: *It's okay, Kim, everything's great!* (Wouldn't that just tick you off even more?!) I would let that go and just embrace a thought like: *I've been in this kind of low state before and found things turned around*, or: *It's okay to just let myself feel this and let the energy move.*

We percolate with the new, slightly higher thought for several seconds—it takes about seventeen seconds to generate that electromagnetic and chemical shift—so we integrate this new frequency. Then we feel slightly different and can begin to move even higher.

I have an example that guides you through doing this exercise for yourself included in your book bonuses.

Go to DrKimD.com/BYOHbonuses to view the video as I guide you in applying this process for yourself.

Once you understand *your attention is your creative power*, do not let it be hijacked. Much around you calls for your attention immediately and hooks you with evidence that the old beliefs are true. Your attention goes to the highest bidder; whoever is being the loudest or most interesting is going to get your attention. But you can consciously choose to *take your attention back* because you always have the ability to change your focus of attention. You get to decide where you put your creative power by deciding where to focus your attention.

The *only* two things you truly have choice about are what you do with your body and where you put your attention, as Londin Angel Winters tells us.

What You Focus On Expands

The first part of cultivating your power to allow instant healing is to realize what you focus on expands. Bring to your awareness a time when you felt amazing. Maybe you were with a lover or a child or doing something you love to do, and time seemed to fly by. Maybe it was a time when you received unexpected news, and it was the greatest news you could've imagined. Maybe it was a peaceful moment with a loved one. Maybe it was time alone in nature where you felt deep joy. Think of a time like this and bring your attention to it. Take several seconds to ponder this with your eyes closed and breathe. Let yourself begin to feel the experience, seeing the sights, hearing the sounds, smelling the scents, feeling the breeze or touch, and tasting the moment. Relax your shoulders as you breathe.

When you do this brief exercise, you immediately shift your electromagnetic field. You shift your vibrational frequency toward the frequency of that experience. That joy, that love, that peace, that excitement, and whatever it was in the experience is recreated here, now, in this moment.

If you practice this over and over, it will consistently bring you into a higher set point for your vibration, a higher set point for what is going on chemically in your body, a higher set point of what is happening neurologically in your brain function, and a higher set point for the way your genes are influenced toward health. As what you focus on expands on a cellular, chemical, and electromagnetic level, it is up to you to cultivate that by harnessing the power of your attention.

You Are in Charge of Where Your Attention Flows

If you understand your attention is your creative power and where you direct your focus expands, of course you want to have the ability to cultivate where you put your attention. That day on the beach when I had the big awakening and finally started really listening to my body was when I began to follow this principle without knowing it. That day, I had a different conversation with my body. I dropped into listening instead of trying to fight my disease and my pain. I decided to be a *receiver* instead of trying to make that experience go away. Instead of the *fearful observer*, noticing the bad things happening and wanting to control them, I entered the *loving observer* who knows she is powerful and it's okay to let the moment in as it is.

This created a new chemistry, a new neurological expression, and a new electromagnetic transmission. That day, my body showed me the awareness of all the ways I was fighting myself. I had been busting my butt to work hard. I had always wanted to do more, to go beyond what I had done before, to constantly improve. I had run a marathon to manage the stress of medical school, but continuing to do it this way was hard on my body. It was time to release the stress rather than manage it. I had learned to push myself to study hard, do well, work out, stay fit, be the best person I could be. My life had become like a never-ending self-improvement program. I realized at the core of this was a feeling of inadequacy and a deep fear of failure. When I dropped in and listened, I realized *fighting* against this belief was exactly what was creating the autoimmune disease. Diagnosis or no diagnosis, my body was reflecting the fight I was in.

The body always reflects the state you are in. It is not that your body is bad or is working against you or is letting you down or you have a disease. It's not that you're being punished for something you did in the past or for not being a better person. Your body is reflecting your electromagnetic state, the consciousness you are in right now.

Have you ever felt like everything is a disaster? Like everything looks and feels miserable and there is no way out?

That's not reality; that's your frequency. When I have moments like that, I realize what's happening and relax my body. The Universe is reflecting my tension and fear. This potent moment—the time that looks and feels like crap!—is my opportunity to transmute the deepest densities arising in my system.

If your body is reflecting fight, tension, and struggle, it is inflamed, in discord and dis-ease, and everything looks like a disaster. Let go. Remember this truth. Breathe. *Do not engage with the disaster.* That's a trap and will just keep it all going.

Now I let all kinds of clusters resolve. I let go and find joy, which may be just choosing to walk away from the situation, get some time with nature, take a nap, or write a love note to myself for encouragement. It always shifts my circumstances and my mind.

Wherever your attention goes is where your energy flows. You are in charge of where your attention goes.

When I finally began to receive my illness as a gift, it was a wake-up call to show me where I had been buying into struggle, lack, and inadequacy that did not even exist. I had been fighting against it, and now I could choose to let go and live in flow. In that flow state, my body worked better, my health accelerated and improved, and I was more likely to succeed. I was more likely to perform well in my exams in medical school. I more easily retained the information I was learning. I had fun. I did not have to be in the fight to succeed. It was exactly that fight creating the problem. It was remarkable that, within days, my symptoms completely resolved.

I had changed the channel consistently enough that I began to reside in this new state all the time. The pain went away. The spasms went away. My joint pain resolved. I was able to start running again. I had energy. I had vitality. My body reflected the health I had put my attention on.

If You Get Hijacked, Life Shows You How to Bring Yourself Back

You will not become a master all at once on this journey to cultivate the power of your attention. You may get hijacked, and it's okay. The point is not *never* getting hijacked and going back to the old programming. The point is lovingly and gently noticing being hijackedand letting it be okay and bringing your attention back into presence. It's pretty much inevitable your energy will get hijacked. Thankfully, you have a built-in system to let you know exactly when it happens.

Your body can live only in the now. It registers the exact moment you've given your power away, bought into the B.S. belief systems again, and started resonating with a lie. Your body is always going to show you when you are in a low-vibrational field. When you are more sensitive, after practicing this work and becoming more skilled at tuning in, you feel that attunement immediately. You may feel the low vibration or heaviness that comes when you have bought into a negative belief. You may feel the tension of a low-frequency dread or fear. You may feel physical fatigue when your mind is ruminating on problems and buying into powerlessness.

Whether you're sensitive and notice the subtle shifts immediately or you're less present to what's happening in you, and you only become aware of the energy after it's physically manifested in symptoms, it's okay. Life is on your side to show you—to get you to tune in and to bring presence *here* so something lighter can manifest.

You are that lightness.

You are that light.

Be here, now, fully with your experience as it is. *That* is the medicine. That is the healing.

Even if you believe you are not very sensitive, your body is always registering the information. It will turn up the volume to get your attention. When the initial, more subtle changes persist, the body will begin to physically manifest this energy to get your attention. You may catch it way upstream when some minor discord arrives, or you may become aware farther downstream when inflammation and physical symptoms have manifested. Even if your DNA has already changed or disease has occurred, you can still reverse the whole process. You do this simply by bringing your attention back to witness and observe what you are experiencing right now.

Don't try to bring your attention to something "positive." This is where most people go wrong. It can be hard to bring your attention to the frequency of: *I am so healthy, everything is perfect* when you feel like absolute crap. So begin by going for something more general and lighter that will stick, like: *It is okay to be feeling the way I am feeling now.* Even though part of you does not want to feel what you are feeling in that moment, and absolutely thinks it is the worst thing in the world, that little bit of acceptance is less resistant than fighting against it and trying to make it change. This is especially important when you feel powerless because a disease has already manifested.

You can generate this shift simply by bringing more presence into your body right now. Soften your body to feel and sense what you are feeling. Drop in and let your shoulders relax, and let your breath come all the way down into your belly. By breathing in a relaxed way, you will sense more than you did just a moment ago. Do not be afraid of what comes up when you do this. You are going to notice everything that has been repressed, which is usually all the unwanted and rejected stuff. You do not have to be afraid because it is all just energy, and energy wants to move.

Emotion is energy in motion. The more you let the energy move, the lighter your emotional state will be. Be willing to accept whatever is right here, right now. Pause, relax your body, take a few breaths, and start to notice. The more you do this, the more attuned your body becomes to the energy field and vibration you are in. Whenever you notice a dense state—whether it is physical, mental, or emotional—bring your awareness back to your breath, sense your body, relax your shoulders, and let your body know it is okay to feel what you feel.

Sensitive people feel a subtle discord in vibration. It may feel like depression, worry, or heaviness. If you are not quite as sensitive, it may already be manifesting emotionally, and you may have more of a chronic depressive state or even an anxiety disorder. Maybe you have a lot of anger and are feeling constantly frustrated. It is okay; welcome that. Maybe you're not as aware emotionally, and you know things are not working out in your life. Welcome whatever you are noticing. You may have shut down your sensitivity and are resisting your emotions. Maybe only the physical manifestation gets your attention. That is okay because it shows you your body is on your side. Your body is reflecting your inner state to give you information and feedback. If you can stay curious, you will tune in and allow the energy to move.

I have seen conditions such as Stage IV cancer, Hashimoto's thyroid disease, inflammatory bowel disease, multiple sclerosis (MS), and all kinds of severe pain syndromes and neurological diseases turn around in a very short time when a person does this work. That is how powerful the electromagnetic shift is on your physical body.

One of the most powerful things you can do if you have manifested discord or disease at the physical level is remember the only reason it is there is to get your attention, so you can make a shift. It is there so you can become more conscious of what you are holding subconsciously and let it go. Discord or disease is there to assist you in getting more present, so you can shift to a higher frequency. In a very small way, perhaps just 2%, allow yourself to receive the disease, illness, or physical symptoms as the gift they are. Even if it does not make sense. Even if you are triggered hearing me say this, *soften your body*. Physically soften your body, relax your shoulders, breathe more fully, and start to let in what this really is—something here to invite you to choose a new way.

YOUR MAP DIRECTLY TO THE ROOT CAUSE

Your body knows exactly what's keeping your illness, symptoms, and challenges in place. When you tune in and listen, it will lead you right to the underlying energy and show you what's required for a resolution.

The wisdom inside your body always knows what is true. Everything you've learned, and in fact, everything contained in all the textbooks and medical journals ever created in the history of the world does not have anything on the wisdom running through your body right now. Everything we think we know is still only an infinitesimally small fraction of everything that the wisdom knows.

The Intelligence that created your body and your systems is moving through you right now. When you tune in and tap into your body and your sensation, and you allow receptivity by softening your body, you let in awareness of that Intelligence.

Your brain waves change dramatically when you simply soften your body, slow your breathing, and bring your attention to sensation. You move from high beta brain waves—which are faster and aligned with memories, programs, and everything you have learned—to low beta brain waves or alpha brain waves, and you become much more receptive to insight and new perception. By shifting your awareness and increasing your attention on your body and your breath, you are changing your brain wave pattern and your electromagnetic field.

Think of the body as a computer system. Your computer has all kinds of programs on it, but if you want to reboot your computer, upload new data, and start working with an updated operating system, you have to shut it off and reboot it.

The same is true in your body. If you are in high beta, you are functioning in your normal reality, playing out the thoughts, ideas, and conclusions you've held from your beliefs and from the past. This conglomerate of programming makes up what I call the *personal self* or the small-self. The more we live from the small-self, the more we keep this programming alive. The personal self has its own level of inflammation and tension in place to keep things together and battle through reality. The personal self will go about life as if *it* is the source of your outcomes, as if it is the cause. It's just the small-self, but it takes on the world, trying to make things happen, trying to get through your day, work hard, and make changes. The more we activate and live through the personal self, the more we keep in place the inflammation, tension, illness, and lack that go along with it. We may pull it off and get through another day, but we can never experience true freedom, well-being, or prosperity through being the personal self. No matter how hard the personal self tries, it cannot get there. That's because identifying as the personal self blocks the Life Force that would allow your body to heal and integrate something new.

You have to hit the pause button, let go of the outside world, let go of doing and trying, and delete the old programs before a new truth can come in. You have to let go of the attachment to making things different first. Turn off your brain and your system so that it can integrate the Higher Intelligence that can heal your body and can heal your life. The willingness to shut off and shut down is the greatest contribution to your health because it will create more for you when you reboot the system. Your computer will work thousands of times faster. There is no point in managing your life from the old programs. You are going to get more out of turning them off and letting your wisdom guide you.

Decode What Your Body Is Telling You

I was recently working with a client named Beth whose healthcare providers had diagnosed her with severe Lyme Disease, chronic fatigue syndrome, and some neurologic symptoms they told her were MS. There were a few other obscure diagnoses that Beth was working with, but no one had been able to help her get better. When we started doing this work, she did not know what was going on within herself. She was at a complete loss as to why her body had become progressively worse and what was at the root of why she hadn't cleared these illnesses.

Beth was experiencing physical symptoms—fatigue, joint pain—as well as anxiety and depression, and she was no longer able to compete in triathlons as she had for years. When we began working together, I guided Beth to drop into her body and let sensation in. At first, this was very unfamiliar; then with practice, it was like a whole universe appeared. She felt many emotions—like fear, powerlessness, and anger—a lot of things that had been underneath the surface of her physical symptoms. There was fear things would get worse. There was anger about not being able to do the things she used to do. There was powerlessness that, after years of dealing with this, nothing was helping, and no matter what she did, she wasn't getting better.

When Beth continued moving into the emotion, letting in sensation and breathing through the energies, a lot of old memories and beliefs came up. She became aware of things that happened in her childhood with her father she had completely blocked out. Beth realized she had never felt safe as a child. Her father hit her when she cried, and there was no space for her to express her emotions. She realized that when she was very young, a small part of her decided to totally shut down so she would not get into trouble, get hurt, or get hit, and she could survive.

Beth followed her symptoms deeper into her emotions, and then followed those emotions into her memories and beliefs. The act of sitting with the emotions, breathing through them, witnessing, and honoring what was there—began clearing things for her; she felt a whole lot lighter.

Beth felt sensations in her body where she was previously numb. When we had started our work, I had asked her to breathe all the way into her pelvis. She had said, "Nothing is happening. I am doing it wrong." When she felt the energy flowing all the way through her body, she could also feel the quality of that energy. If she was in that self-denial and repression program, subconsciously thinking about her own powerlessness, she would sense that immediately in her body. She could feel the heaviness. She could feel the fear arise. Instead of holding that repression, she could let it shift. In the weeks of working together, she continued this practice, letting her body know: *It is okay to feel what you feel*—reversing the programs introduced when she was a child, and which she had been taught to hold in.

Beth began unwinding that pattern and letting her body release. Sometimes she released the energy by making sounds as she exhaled. Sometimes the energy was released by moving. As the energy began to release, her physical symptoms and all the "diseases" began to resolve. Her body cleared the Lyme infection, and she has regained her energy and begun enjoying activities again.

Even if you think you do not know what is underneath your symptoms, you can bring presence, soften your body, and drop in, and your body will show you. Your body will release your conflict and dis-ease. It knows how to do that.

Authority: Who Are You Letting Be the Author of Your Life?

I often see patients who have been given a diagnosis buy into all the ideas, beliefs, and assumptions the diagnosis is supposed to mean. They think they *have to* be on medication. They think they will get progressively worse. They think there is something wrong with them and their body is broken. That diagnosis is packaged with the idea of what is going to happen next, why it happened in the first place, what went wrong, and what they need to do now.

None of those things may be in any way true on any level. We give our power away to our practitioner who says: *There is nothing that can be done*, or says, *You will always have to be on medication*, or says, *You have XYZ disease and, therefore, you need this treatment.*

Without even thinking, we assume that to be true. All the while, our cells are listening, so we get on the program of that "truth" and are going to live it out. That disease program is going to play out in our body because we're giving it our energy and attention.

But what if when you're given a diagnosis or the opinion of a doctor, you were to just observe what's happening and feel into that moment, as I did? What does it feel like to take on those ideas and buy into that reality? Light or heavy?

I felt very heavy. I felt like I was going to die. I wanted to quit everything. When I realized: *Wait a minute—what if this is not true for me*, I immediately felt light and powerful. That is when my body began healing. I was no longer on the program of my doctor's perspective, I was no longer on the program of: *There's something wrong with me*, and I got back into alignment with the truth of my own inner knowing.

You can do the same thing. Look at how you feel about the medications you are on, the treatments you are on, the supplement regimen you are on, and the diet regimen you are on.

What is your perspective? Is it heavy? Is it light?

Maybe it is life-giving. Maybe you feel amazing and grateful you have life-giving solutions working for you. You are moving forward. Things are speeding up. Resources are coming in. That will feel light. Let that strengthen you. Receive it all.

But maybe it is the opposite, and you feel uncertain or afraid. You see things getting worse and worse, and you are worried. That is a sure indicator your attention got hijacked, and you are giving your power away to the limiting beliefs. You are giving your authority away, and you are buying into a program not true for you.

I often see overwhelm in the patients and clients I work with when they are trying to heal themselves. They will learn everything they can, read dozens of books, or work with a bunch of coaches or experts. Maybe there is a rigid diet regimen they have adopted, or maybe there is a complicated supplement regimen, and they are overwhelmed. I call it out.

It can be confusing because they think: *Aren't these things supposed to be good for me?*

"I don't know," I'll tell them, "Let's look; let's feel it out. Let's tune into what is true for you now that will create the highest possibility. Until you release the assumptions you have about those approaches, you will not know."

To get that clarity, you've got to release the mind with all its ideas, conclusions, and assumptions and drop into the body. When you find you are in overwhelm, soften your body so your awareness can be more fully present. Use it as an opportunity to develop some awareness. First, notice you are operating in a system that is not your truth. It may be your mom's belief system saying, "As you get older you have to fight harder for your health. You have to work at it, or it will all fall apart."

It may be your father's belief system saying, "Keep working and pull yourself up by the bootstraps. Keep pushing hard to overcome things. Grit your teeth and march your way through it."

That is fine and that may have worked for them, but is it working for you to live in the robust health of joy and aliveness you are here to live?

If it is not, dump it. You do not need to live in someone else's belief system.

Your wisdom always shows you when you are doing this; it is when you feel *overwhelmed*. You will feel heavy with a sense of dread. That is a sure indicator you are not operating according to *your* truth. Even the belief system that says *your body is a physical, solid, separate thing* can make things impossible. Buying into that belief is going to be super heavy for a lot of people because in that realm and perspective of reality there are not resources to match what you desire and are ready to receive. You want to feel great now. You want to feel light and be free, to have unconditional self-expression, acceptance, love, and joy. That is not going to happen in a system claiming you are broken, and telling you to be on medication with lots of side effects that are killing you. Being free does not exist in that system. You have to release the whole foundation of that belief system and remember: *I am pure energy. My body and life can instantaneously shift to life in light, freedom, and Truth.*

Truth with a capital "T" is something that is true whether you believe it or not. It is nature. It is operating whether you subscribe to it or not. It is universally true.

When you get on the track of Truth, you are going to know what is right for you. It feels light when you consider it because it's True. The Truth will set you free. When you are asked, "Would you like to go to lunch on Friday?" you don't automatically respond with what the programming says you *should* do. We don't go into the behavior of a "good girl" or "good boy" who is compliant and does what they are told. We don't play out the program unconsciously. When you get on the track of Truth, you are aware. You feel your heart's desire, and you sense either a "yes" or a "no thank you" depending on what's True and in your highest interest.

If you stay in the mind—which is the *protective personality*, the fight or flight nervous system is activated and you stay in the programs. You don't feel the innate heart's desire. You cannot see beyond what you believe and what you have been taught. In that case, nothing I am saying will make any sense. Or maybe you understand it cognitively, but you haven't yet integrated it on a cellular level. When you're in the mind, with the programs running, you are not receptive to anything new. If you soften your body, that alone allows some of those perspectives to release. Softening your body allows your system to be more receptive to new perspectives and higher Intelligence. It takes courage to do this because we hold to a lot of beliefs we think are true and will protect us. If we soften our body, relax, slow down, and breathe more deeply, we let go of some of those protections—the protections that say *keep going, tighten up, don't stop, don't look up.*

You must have courage and trust enough to open up and get curious instead of clamping down and fighting. I am asking a lot here, but the promise is that this allows you to leverage the Universe. This is how your electromagnetic nervous system works. This is how the technology and the wisdom of your body works. You can absolutely trust what happens when you pause, tune in, and honor your truth.

Go to Your Heart for Answers, Not the Program

Another sure indicator you are living in a limited belief system, paradigm, or foundation of reality that is not your Truth is when you're challenged and can see no solutions. You do not have an answer, there are no possibilities, and it looks like something needs to happen and there is no way it can happen.

There's only one way to open things up; it has to start within you. Drop in and feel the heaviness of what you're facing, fully registering the moment without resistance. Registering the heaviness is a gift because that is your receptivity to your wisdom, which is showing you this a lie. Your body is going to register truth or lie as lightness or heaviness. Tuning in allows you to sense the moment and to feel the communication from your system. Your wisdom always shows you what you need to see.

A feeling of lightness is always a sign you are moving in the right direction. A feeling of fear is just evidence you are clamped down in fight-or-flight and are in the program. Wisdom never communicates with you through fear. Fear is the programming trying to help you survive, but it's not the Truth. Clamping down, tensing up, and trying to control your reality are not actually going to assist your survival. Softening assists you to let in the moment more fully. That's when Life Force comes in and can create solutions for you. Life is never going to signal you through fear as a way to bring you onto the right path. Fear is always "False Evidence Appearing Real." Your wisdom will inspire you to move onto the right path. It will call you through clarity, desire, and inspiration. These are not the same frequency as fear.

If you tune in, sense your body, and sense whether you feel heavy or light, you will always have the awareness of whether you are on your true path. Following the program will only lead to more lack and limitation, more illness and inflammation, more stuff going wrong to deal with, and more contraction in your life.

Your nature is expansion. When you soften and let Life in, things expand.

Many clients have asked me, "What if something really is wrong? Won't I overlook that if I just soften and relax and do nothing?"

Here's something I will state that you can take to heart, that you can remember each time triggers hook you into the fear programming:

There is nothing wrong.

The idea that something is wrong is the first myth keeping us stuck in the loop of fear. Seeing things as wrong is just a way the ego-mind keeps you looped into the fear programming.

The second big myth that loops us into the fear programming is the idea softening to let in the moment means ignoring things and doing nothing.

It's a lie. When you're more aware and more tuned in, are you more or less likely to respond appropriately? Are you more or less resourced with energy to follow through with that response? Are you more or less clear about what the best response is?

Softening into the moment, surrendering control, actually gives you more power.

That's because when we are in the parasympathetic state—open, soft, receptive—we are always more responsive, more energized, more resourced, and more clear. Always.

We'll also see it's not the small-self doing the responding. It's the *I AM* self, the True Self, the Life Force living through us and guiding us.

You really can trust this Life Force that created you to take care of everything and anything that may be presenting itself in the moment. This is called surrender, and it is the doorway to becoming free from everything that would otherwise haunt you for life.

If you are in a situation where it seems there are no answers or possibilities, or the answers presenting themselves are a nightmare in and of themselves, don't buy it. Soften. You're in a program. Just like when I was told I had to take a lot of medications, change my environment, and never run again. It felt like a death sentence, not a solution. The *solution* was just as bad as the disease. Until we change our frequency, we can't experience something higher. It may look like a solution, but it's not actually an improvement in the overall quality of life.

It's at the same frequency. True solutions do not lie in the same frequency as the problem.

A well-known saying is that we cannot solve a problem from the same consciousness within which it was created. This means we must shift our frequency and consciousness first.

If you tune in and feel the remedy is just as bad or worse than the disease, you can be assured you are operating in a belief system not true for you, and it is time to upgrade. Open to allow it in.

Take a few deep breaths and bring your attention to your heart. This will shift your electromagnetic field. Your heart has receptors called *sensory neurites*, which register a different kind of Intelligence. Unlike your brain, which is a dual organ, pre-programmed to look for threats and go toward the good thing or away from the bad thing—your heart is a singular, non-dual organ and registers unity consciousness. It allows a higher perception of Truth that goes beyond duality and the perception of right and wrong.

Your brain-mind can only register duality; it cannot know Truth. Your heart-mind can be receptive. Your heart can receive information and Intelligence that goes way beyond what your mind can know. It goes beyond what the programs can tell you. You will access wisdom that goes far beyond every medical textbook ever written. You will know what exactly is required for you to heal.

Will you open to your heart? It requires you to have an intention beyond the fear. It takes courage. *Coeur*, from the French, meaning "heart."

Are you ready to let in courage so this can be easy for you? So that your desire to live as love is bigger than your fear?

You can tune into the Intelligence through the heart by just listening and asking questions, softening the body so you are a better receiver.

Daily Integration Exercise 2: Access Innate Intelligence by Connecting to Your Heart

- Relax your shoulders and take slow deep breaths. Let your eyes close and feel your spine straight.

- Bring your attention to the area around your heart. You can place your hands over your heart area if you like.

- Breathe as if it is your heart that's breathing the breath in and out. See the heart area expand out with the inhales. See it let go of everything on the exhales.

- Ask yourself: *What would be the most beneficial thing I could do to bring health and vitality into my life right now?* You can also ask more specifically: *What would strengthen my relationship? What would bring in more wealth and freedom?*

- The awareness will come in when it comes in. It may at first just be a feeling of lightness and relief. There may later be total clarity either through someone telling you the exact right thing at the right time, or a sudden epiphany as you're going about your day where it just hits you.

- Stay present and connected to your heart throughout the day.

Use this as your five-times-a-day exercise as you continue to read this book.

There is a meditation for this in the audios included with this book. DrKimD.com/BYOHbonuses

Each time you do this exercise, you activate the Intelligence of your heart. It activates the receptivity in your nervous system and increases your electromagnetic frequency.

The electromagnetic frequency of the heart is more powerful than that of the brain. This means when you center your attention on your heart, you allow a recalibration and a repatterning of the brain, the nervous system, the immune system, the endocrine system (hormones), and all other areas of the body. The powerful signals radiating through the heart when you connect this way activate all other areas to align with Truth.

Let go of what you know, what you have learned, what the most intelligent doctor on the planet says. *Your* wisdom is the number one expert on everything about *you*. Your wisdom knows the best thing you could possibly eat for lunch today that will support you in being clear and energized in the afternoon. Your wisdom knows if there is a particular food you need to avoid to help release your symptoms. Your wisdom knows the right practitioner to see to be vibrantly healthy. Your wisdom knows the people in your life who strengthen your prosperity and those who weaken it. The more you tune into the heart, the more you become receptive to this information. When you are challenged, when life feels like a conundrum, when things feel impossible, remember—go to your heart. You will activate the electromagnetics and even if you do not figure anything out or consciously get any answers, you have already changed your world. Completely unexpected solutions can arise. Physical ailments can dissolve out of nowhere.

I was once seated next to a woman at dinner who told me her mother-in-law had been recently diagnosed with Stage IV cancer. Her family members were so worried and scared they did not know what to do. She started crying, and I immediately tuned into the awareness of what was going on and asked myself, *"What needs to happen here?"* I had complete and utter clarity this was *not* Stage IV cancer. "She is not going to die," I told her. "I don't know exactly what is going on, but your mother-in-law is going to live a very long life." I didn't know why I was telling her that, and part of me hesitated in case I was mistaken, but the clarity was so strong I shared it all. I found the courage to share because I knew it was true.

Months later I ran into her in town, and she told me that the week after we'd initially met, she learned her mother-in-law had been misdiagnosed. She had osteoporosis, not cancer at all, let alone Stage IV metastatic cancer. With treatment she would go on to live a long and happy life. All was well, but she asked me how I got that awareness at the dinner. In the paradigm of: *I am a physical solid separate thing*, I could not possibly know something like that. Even with all the information from all the medical books ever written, this could not be known. But in the paradigm of *I am pure energy; infinite Intelligence moves through me*, I tuned into the heart, which is a space of love and compassion. I connected with that Intelligence and information, and it was unquestioningly clear. We all have this ability when we tune in. We sometimes just need the courage to ask, to receive, and to let ourselves share.

If you are willing to let go of the foundation of the reality you thought was true and have the courage to venture into something way more expansive, you are going to access unthinkable possibilities, unthinkable miracles. Diagnoses will resolve out of thin air and problems will go away like they did for this woman. We can let the solutions come in *through* us; they do not have to come *from* us. You may not receive information distinctly; you may feel a sense of calm and ease. Follow that; stay in *calm and ease*. You may find there is a spontaneous resolution to your problem.

Or you may be delighted when some weird, obscure, amazing remedy you have never heard of crosses your path. How they come to you is irrelevant; true solutions exist and will be readily available. They will be light, accessible, and have the impact your heart desires.

In the next chapter, you will connect with the truth in your heart. Unlike the mind, the heart will bring you beyond the programming to connect with your true nature for guidance. This is a portal to your Divinity, allowing in possibilities beyond what you have imagined or could ever have created from the small-self.

Are you ready to set yourself free?

CHAPTER FOUR

Your Truth Is Written on Your Heart

If you're going to cultivate your creative power for instant healing and master the ability to focus your attention, it is essential that you center yourself in your heart instead of in the programming. Your space of BE-ing is what sets the stage for everything happening in your body and within your electromagnetic field. So, will you be the space and consciousness of the program—and continue to live in limitation, lack, and fear—or will you be the space and consciousness of Source? You get to choose, and in this chapter you'll see that everything that happens is assisting you in making that choice.

For many people with a chronic illness, dealing with the illness starts to take over their lives. They begin to think it is the worst thing that has ever happened, and they just want to get rid of it. They'll think if only they could get their health back, everything would be so much better. Often, they will come to me and say: *Just make my pain tolerable so I can get on with my life*, or *I just wish I had my energy back*. I commonly hear clients say, "I used to have health. I used to be happy. I used to be active. I want my old life back." They think their illness is a curse or a punishment or, at the very least, an inconvenience. They think: *Let's get this over with, solve the problem, and get on with life.*

Something much deeper is happening, though, and universally I have found when people get underneath their illness and the emotional and mental components creating it, we see there are much bigger issues in their system. The illness is the tip of the iceberg. Once they realize this and have a resolution on a deeper level, they understand something bigger was happening. They receive a gift they didn't realize was there all along.

It isn't possible to simply knock out the pain and continue with everyday life. Something deeper is taking place, and it's happening *for* you. After doing this work and witnessing the real resolution, clients tell me: *I had no idea life could be like this. I am a different person. I am living at a deeper level. I have more compassion for who I am. I have awakened beyond my deepest pains and deepest fears and let all of that go. I am more whole than I ever imagined I could be.*

Doing this work creates something infinitely more magnificent than getting rid of disease and marching on with life in your same old consciousness. It ends up creating such a profound shift for a person that they are forever changed in the best possible way. Through courage, they begin to see their illness is bringing them through a journey to go deeper into themselves. The purpose of this journey is not freeing yourself from illness alone, but also becoming more of who you are, so the problem can dissolve. The illness is the space holder for something much deeper within you that's ready to resolve. This core issue is coming up to be released.

The real process unfolds when you look at what's underneath your symptoms, and the magnificence of who you are becomes apparent. When you are faced with something unwanted, it is not an obstacle to overcome or an inconvenience to deal with. It is a deeper truth you are meant to integrate. When you are faced with what you do *not* want, you are being invited into more of what you *do* want. This expansion is your heart's deepest desire.

You are here to awaken to the truth, not to put a bandage over the falsehood you are carrying around. You will realize your experience is not a solitary experience of going through an illness; it is a collective experience of all of us awakening. We are leaving behind separation consciousness—the idea that: *I am a separate solid self, distinct from everyone else,* and we enter unity consciousness. *I am pure energy. I am an infinite being having a physical experience. I am connected with everyone and everything. I am part of Creator. I am powerful.* We enter the realm of the True Self. Understanding this through the mind is just more B.S. The way we access, feel, and integrate this is through the heart.

When you drop into the heart, which is the main electromagnetic center of the body, and come out of the mind and the programming, you register the truth. You register Divine Intelligence. You register your true desires instead of the programming. You register who you really are.

The experience of having an illness or problem that won't go away no matter what you do calls you deeper into yourself to let go of everything you've been holding. Because what you already know is not "working," it invites you to allow a major change and a shift within yourself. When you receive your experiences instead of resisting them by trying to fix, avoid, or escape them, you enter more and more into surrender. This brings you into your True Self.

When you surrender, your body is no longer being overstimulated with the fear programs of the false-self. It gets a break. Regeneration can then happen. When you live from your True Self, you align with Source and powerful healing comes in. This greatly benefits your body. You are now sourcing your body from Source Consciousness, and you will see issues resolve.

It also benefits everyone around you because you are one more person awakening out of the program of collective consciousness and popping into truth. You are awakened and you are also an awakener. Your body and your electromagnetic system function on a higher level and will call everyone else into that same functionality. An awakened person wakes others up too. You see life is meant to be a gift, and you can live your magnificence through all the experiences and challenges you are having.

YOUR HEART LEADS THE WAY

You may have bought into the programming that says: *Your inner world is worthless, Your outer achievements are your only real value, There is nothing happening within you,* and *If you overcome that worthlessness and prove yourself, you may get somewhere in life.* It is easy to get disconnected from what you know deep within your heart when society reflects these programs. You may have found yourself thinking: *I don't know what I want* or *I don't know what I am passionate about,* because you've become so accustomed to what you are supposed to do and who you are supposed to be, you've stopped tuning into your inner voice. The brain stops paying attention to the more essential, big-picture information like: *What is my heart's deepest desire? What do I truly care about? What lights me up? How much fun could I have right now?*

You always have that awareness somewhere within you. It's just a matter of nurturing it rather than squashing it. Notice whether you are doing this. When something inspires you and you think: *Oh my gosh, this would be amazing!* and it is quickly followed by: *Yeah, but that will never work because . . .*

When you do this, you are overriding your passion and inner knowing of what would make you more alive. You are squashing awareness of what brings you joy in favor of what you think is true, which is the programming. You think the program is the truth and your dreams are unrealistic or irresponsible.

If your end outcome is survival, this may seem like a good idea. You sacrifice real joy or aliveness, but at least you're still here. However, it's an illusion. The very thing you think ensures your survival is actually killing you. The program doesn't work to enhance survival *or* to create a life of joy. It just keeps you on the hamster wheel *thinking* you're getting somewhere. When you look at others who are living according to the program, you would be hard-pressed to find anyone emanating pure joy or living in robust aliveness. Living the program is not going to create true wealth, health, joy, or gratitude, no matter how long you keep at it. You may think it is unrealistic to live in joy, so you quiet down the inner calling rather than question the program.

But what if your experiences are calling your attention to where you got it wrong? When your challenge or illness is not resolving, no matter what you do, and the more you fight it, the more persistent those challenges become, those experiences are showing you where you made a faulty conclusion and that it's time to let it go.

What if your greatest challenges are ultimately an invitation to let go of everything you think is true, and tune into that calling within your heart to navigate your reality and your choices? Are you ready to live your life from an entirely different premise?

I invite you to consider the truth that your life is meant to be a magnificent work of art. No matter how it's gone up until now, it really is all a part of that masterpiece. From wherever you are, you can tune in and start allowing that expansion. You are free to follow your heart and choose your highest path. When you do, your life expands in abundance. This benefits you and it benefits everyone. You are not separate. Unlike choosing what's best for your small-self ego, choosing from your heart is a gift to all the world. Everyone benefits whether they know it or not. You expand in courage, love, and power, and everyone benefits.

How do you tune in and start that path? Your heart, the electromagnetic center of your body, is your area of receptivity to all of it. In any moment, you can clearly see your highest path, the choices bring you more abundance, and the awareness of what your heart's desires are.

Why Your Bliss Seems Too Good to Be True

If anything I have said resonates with you, brings a sense of lightness, or percolates an effervescent sensation within your body, it is because it's resonating with something awakening within *you*. Part of you knows this deep Divine Truth, and it is starting to wake up and express itself even more fully. There may also be doubt arising from what I've shared here, and you may think: *Yeah maybe for other people but not for me*, or *Maybe for Kim because she is XYZ, but not for me because I do not have those traits or characteristics*. Or you think: *You can't have it all; there has to be some compromise in life*. You buy into those doubts and limitations because that is what you have been taught.

Is everyone around you living some form of limitation and lack, trying to tell you *that is the way life is* and you'd better get used to it?

They'll tell you to be careful; you need to be responsible because reaching for real joy is wrong and will put you at risk. It's a lie. Living the program makes you dead even before you die. When you are instead willing to prioritize your true passions and take full responsibility for everything in your life, you allow for magnificent change. You allow massive change to take place because everything is happening as an expression and reflection of where you put your energy; it is a reflection of your own beliefs and inner choices, whether they are conscious or unconscious. When you look at life as an invitation to go within, you immediately start letting go of things that are not serving you.

Let's say you are in a relationship or relationships that are not so great. Maybe other people have lots of expectations of you; you have lots of obligations to them; you are not having a lot of fun; you are not fully expressed; you are not deeply in joy and love. There is limitation in those relationships. Maybe you do not feel fully accepted so you hold things in and do not let people know how you feel. Maybe you feel judged, so you pretend to be someone you are not. This is going to cause deep pain.

If you drop into your body, you will feel a heaviness, a pit in your stomach, or a pressure on your chest. If you drop in, you are going to realize what you are doing to yourself. By witnessing all of this and just feeling that heaviness in your chest or that pit in your stomach as you breathe, you can shift these energies in your body. That will then shift all your relationships. If your relationship had shown up as perfect before you made this inner shift, you would never access those spaces within your own energy system. Healing would never happen because you would stay clueless about what was inside you. Continuing to suppress your emotions would suck away your Life Force and deplete your health, but you would be at a loss because you'd have no idea those energies were even in there, and you'd be powerless to do anything about them.

This is where most people reside when they keep shutting down their emotions.

But life is on your side. It is calling you into your magnificent alignment, creation, and light. It's bringing all of this up to your awareness. You can receive that enlightenment and let it in. You can realize you are only suffering because you are buying into a lie. You can make a new choice. You will see you have bought into the idea you are not worthy of having a great relationship or, like I did for so long, buy into the belief *I'm no prize package so I should be abused.* You may believe a great relationship does not exist, so you settle for what you get.

If you live that program out and ignore what you feel, you may think *this is just the way things are.* But if you drop into the body, soften, and welcome more presence, what you are feeling cannot be ignored. That is when you gain real power and real leverage to breathe into those sensations, to soften those areas where you feel the heaviness, or the fluttering, or the pressure, and let your breath come more fully into those areas. This is how the energy is released.

You must drop into your body, bring your presence into your body here now, to shift this programming. This is what you are doing through the Daily Integration Exercises.

If you welcome what you notice and breathe, you witness the energy dissipate, it dissolves and is no longer being maintained in your system. It is only what you resist that persists. If you are not suppressing it, it dissolves. That is when you notice new sensations and new possibilities. Relationships transform, amazing people come into your life, or someone who has always treated you badly suddenly treats you very lovingly and with kindness.

Maybe you never met an available partner. All of a sudden, someone enters your life who would have previously seemed too good to be true. You're able to let them in because you have made space for that experience. Now you get to have a partnership and have an available person who is interested in you and devoted to you. You can allow something you had previously blocked out or pushed away because you had thought it was impossible.

The same is true with your health, money, or career. If you look at the movie screen of what is showing up in your life and you drop into the moment, how do you feel?

What is the actual *experience* compared to what you think is going on?

When you let the moment in, you sense, feel, and connect with the energy. You can tense and resist to protect yourself from it, or you can let it in and let the transmutation happen. You can choose to bring your presence to that sensation and to that experience. You can bring your breath to that sensation and that experience. That presence is the healer. You allow the energy to move and release so something new can manifest.

Do you think something seems too good to be true when you feel that inner yearning for expansion?

When your inner self says: *Yes, oh my gosh this will be amazing!* do you then have the belief: *Oh, forget it; that won't happen?* If something amazing comes into your life, are you afraid it won't last?

That is because you are harboring beliefs you cannot have the things you desire, that you are not good enough for them. Maybe you even believe you shouldn't want them.

Remember it is only your beliefs in the way; your doubts and self-talk are not reality. If your heart is yearning for a healthier body, more energy, or full resolution of an illness—it is not a pipe dream. You're not making it up. Your natural state is to be in joy, passionately alive. Your dreams are written on your heart. They will always call out to you. Let them in. The underlying energy of freedom and vitality are available right here, right now, and do not require something to happen first.

Don't Wait for Joy

What if you let energy, passion, and joy in as if you are living that experience right now? This is what ignites cellular change. It allows a higher electromagnetic expression to percolate through your body and allows you to see possibilities you could not have seen before. You will witness those synchronicities lead to a resolution which would not have happened otherwise.

Many clients say, "Once my body heals, I'll be happy and joyful." They're waiting for the result to show up first. It can't. If you think it's impossible for you to feel a little lighter, a little freer, before things shift physically, you will never get there.

Whether a man thinks he can or cannot, he is right.
~ Henry Ford.

The key to physical manifestation lies within your thinking. Don't let those beliefs get in the way. Choose to let yourself feel 2% more well right now. The body will follow.

Do not require your physical health to already be better before you start to let yourself feel lighter. It is the sensation of lightness that activates your electromagnetic field and lets the physical healing begin.

Your Heart's Desires Call You to Your True Self

Your heart is never going to let you down. It does not suddenly put something in your head that is unattainable or impossible. It does not dangle a possibility in front of your nose that is not ready for you to access, like some cruel cosmic game. The electromagnetics of the heart register awareness, sensation, possibilities, ideas, and inspirations that are *here now* in your energy field, available to you. Are they *accessible*? That is up to you. Open.

Maybe you are about to meet the love of your life. That person exists, and it is only a matter of time, navigating the right pieces of the puzzle, and that person will cross paths with you. Or it may only be a matter of a few synchronicities before you land your ideal job or career or receive unthinkable amounts of money. The mind would never know that is possible. It cannot know an ideal partner just moved to your town, and if you go to your neighborhood coffee shop, you are going to meet them on Monday at two o'clock in the afternoon. But the heart can navigate your now moment to bring those exact kinds of things about. If you tune into the heart and feel inspired to go get a cup of coffee *right now*, do it. Maybe you meet your greatest partner, get married, and live a long life together. Maybe you meet a business collaborator who changes your life. Everything is possible. When you follow your heart, amazing things happen.

When you are not tuned into those sensations because you are plugged into the program, you either do not feel any calling or you override it with excuses: *I can't go now. My life is not going to work if I do not put my nose to the grindstone and get this done right now or I can't afford to do that.* Perhaps you start to follow an action by making a choice to buy a new course that can change your life. Then you rethink: *Oh no, no, no—I made the wrong decision. That is irresponsible. I need to get my money back.* Either way, it is always a choice.

That choice is either in service to the heart . . . or is a slave to the mind. Let the inner wisdom lead your choices, behaviors, and actions. Or continue to override them because you buy into the fear program and give it your energy and let that guide your choices, actions, and behaviors. Either way, you win. The former will show you the power in you; the latter will bring you more clarity that following fear always leads to greater contraction and lack.

One client I worked with, Sheri, had chronic fatigue syndrome and multiple other diagnoses. She was teaching full time and was desperate to get out . . . but didn't see a way. "In twelve years, I can retire and have a stipend for life," she rationalized. She was pushing herself every day to endure—*for twelve years!*—something she dreaded.

I asked her if she was willing to consider that this illness was her body letting her know staying on that path was not the best way. Sheri seemed terrified. "But I have to do this. I can't just do what my body wants; I have to make money."

I asked her, "Do you really believe the Infinite Intelligence that created you is overlooking the fact that having your bills taken care of is a necessary part of the equation?"

I invited her to let go of all the beliefs and fears around money and career, and open to trust. Many tears and shaking came. What unearthed was a deep-seated terror after being raised in a family where emotions were not recognized and where outer success was the only thing deemed important.

"I never realized I felt this way. I never cry. I am not an emotional person," Sheri said, apologizing profusely. I invited her to let go of all the ideas she had about who she is. More tears and more shaking followed, and then a full surrender, softening of her body, and wailing.

When this slowed, she was breathing fully and was glowing.

"That felt amazing." she shared. Sheri began to feel all kinds of things, especially a strong sense of confidence and an inspiration to start her own private tutoring services for kids. She had been hesitant about leaving the school system before, but now she said, "They don't own me. I am talented and can do whatever I want. I'll keep listening and let my heart show me."

Sheri got all her energy back, healed from the other illnesses, and began a new business teaching on her own.

Your heart's desires are not tuning you into some unrealistic pipe dream. They bring you into alignment with your True Self, into alignment with the experiences, people, and situations that are your organically best matches. Your heart can align you with your highest fulfillment like a job or an opportunity. Your heart can align you with the resources and ideas to fuel an amazing project. You can trust and let in the resources for all your greatest inspirations. But you must open to realize life is on your side, and it's okay to let go.

This relates directly to your health. When you make the choices that make your heart sing, bring you your greatest joy, and lead you to greater fulfillment, those are the very choices that most support, nurture, and nourish your health and body. More important than eating the right food or going all-organic or raw vegan, or anything you do that you think would contribute to your health, the number one thing that lights your body up, makes your cells sing, reverses cellular disease, detoxifies your body, activates the most favorable gut microbiome, and has your body be fully alive, reversing deterioration instead of accelerating it—is living in alignment with your True Self. That is the Fountain of Youth.

A lot of people ask me, "What do you do to stay so fit and healthy? Are you running, are you doing yoga, are you eating a certain way? I want to do whatever you are doing."

I have been shown this truth for years because I have committed to living my truest self and to allowing my authentic expression:

- I do not have a strict regimen of diet or exercise.

- If something is a *no*, I honor that. If something is a *yes*, I honor that.

- If there is something to be said, I find a way to say it.

- If a relationship feels discordant, I have a conversation to resolve it, or I let that relationship go.

- If something feels inorganic or inauthentic in my work or business, I make a revision, so I am no longer involved with it.

- I don't make commitments that do not feed me and fuel me, that do not feel right in my heart.

- I allow fluidity and expression to be the #1 priority, so the energy currents are open, and energy is coursing freely through my being.

I think that last item—more than any physical thing I have ever done or ever could do— is what contributes to my level of health, well-being, resilience, and vitality.

The sensory neurites of your heart are registering what is already here in this moment as a possibility for you. It is not registering your hopes: *Oh, I wish that could be, but it is probably not going to happen,* or unrealistic dreams: *I wish someday this could happen.* You would not have that desire and calling for something that does not already exist as a possibility, because if it were not here now, there would be nothing to spark that *yes* and spark inspiration and desire. If you can even imagine your ideal career and how it would feel, not necessarily the specifics of it, but even just the generality like: *It would be awesome to do something that inspires me, to be doing something I care about that makes a real contribution in the world*—that is enough for you to know something else is available.

Many people experience this in the opposite way. The heart registers the new possibilities and is speaking to them, but instead of feeling that inspiration, they become aware of the desperation. Because they're closing to the heart, they feel the heaviness of staying where they are, the dread of continuing one more day on the old path. Most don't realize what it means, and they let it strengthen the old belief they'll never get what they want. But the dread of staying where you are is another sure sign your heart is registering new possibilities now available to you. One hundred percent of the time, this dread is an indicator something else has become available. *Ding! Ding! Ding!* your order is up. It is time to make a change and move from where you are.

Way back when I was working in the ER, it became apparent it was time to leave. It was not where I was meant to be. I had known a residency in emergency medicine was part of the equation for me. It deeply strengthened my ability to be in flow during very intense situations and to trust my intuition and act on it, but I also knew it was not the endpoint. After a couple of years of practicing full-time in the ER, it began to weigh heavily on me that nothing else was happening. I started getting anxious.

I thought: *What do I need to do? How do I change my life? I will knock on doors; I will find an opportunity. I will open an osteopathic practice. I will do whatever I have to do. I will figure this one out.*

There was a sense of urgency and desperation. Whenever I tuned into my wisdom, I immediately sensed an inner voice that would tell me: *Be still and know. There is nothing to do. It is all coming for you. It is all happening.* I would immediately feel a sense of peace and calm and continue in my day.

Weeks later, I would feel the same rush of: *Oh my gosh, I can't stand it here. I need a change; there has to be something else. What should I do? What should I do?* and start thinking the same thing: *Let me go knock on doors and find a place to practice the way I want to. Let me get out of here. Let me make my life change. Let me do something different.*

When I would tune into my body and take a few breaths, I would feel again: *Be anxious for nothing, it is all happening for you. Everything is taken care of.* Immediately I would feel a sense of peace. After a while, I began to doubt: *It's not happening. How could it happen? Is it ever really going to happen? Am I stuck here?*

Then something in me would feel the heaviness and know it was not true at all. I would let go immediately and return to a sense of peace. All my doubts and fears came up like this on an almost daily basis. *Was I crazy to think I could do things differently?* It was a difficult, lonely, and uncertain time.

Within a few months of opening, asking for something to come in, and being patient, I spoke with one of my colleagues with whom I had done my osteopathic medicine fellowship. She had gone on to an osteopathic residency. She had a holistic practice focused on how the body heals itself, and she was living a totally different lifestyle. I imagined she was living a fulfilling and amazing life doing what she loved, and I wished I could be doing that too. I felt so frustrated: *Why did I not do that kind of residency training? Why did I not go down that path?*

That would have made it all good. Why did I take this path? What was I thinking? Maybe I did the wrong thing.

But I stayed in my moment. We spoke on the phone, and she told me about her life and said she bought Greg Thompson's practice. Greg was a doctor and mentor of mine in medical school. He was an amazing healer and osteopath I deeply admired. He had a prominent practice adjacent to a large home where he lived with his wife and five children. I wondered: *Where the heck did he go if she bought his practice?* She explained that he had moved to Tennessee to start a new osteopathic medical school.

Suddenly I felt *Ding! Ding! Ding!* lighting me up inside. I thought: *I am not far from Tennessee. I could drive a couple of times a week and be part of the school.* I knew they would love to have me teach there because I had done a lot of teaching in that field: *This would be amazing. I could pop up a couple of times a week and have that layer of meaning I'd been looking for.* I asked my colleague how I could get in touch with him and felt a speeding up: *I have got to get in touch with this guy.*

Within two days I got a call from Greg asking, "What do we need to do to get you up here?!" It turned out the osteopathic medical school was more than four hours away from where I was living in Atlanta—not a hop, skip, and jump. I could not casually transition myself and hold together my life in Atlanta while I did this cool new thing. I would have to make a major change. *I would have to leave everything behind.*

This brought some fear: *Wait a minute—I am in an awesome townhouse in the center of Atlanta. I am living a super cool life.*

I have so many friends; we are always having fun; I can go out any time I want and I make lots of money in the ER. Do I want to give this up? Am I sure about this? I immediately felt an overwhelming sense of certainty: *Kim, this is your moment, let go and move forward.* Even though my mind was suddenly making my current situation sound good, I knew it was time to leave. I felt so enthusiastic, I called a real estate agent before I even checked out the school for an interview. Within about a week and a half, I had driven up to Tennessee, looked at real estate, interviewed, and knew my life was about to change. I sold my house, left my career in the ER, moved to rural Tennessee, and started teaching in the medical school.

In a way, it seemed like I was giving something up, but during those next few months of transition, the time could not pass quickly enough because I knew it was the right thing. It was an acceleration. It was the fulfillment I was yearning for, and it resonated in every part of my being. By following my heart and becoming aware of the discord, I tuned into the possibility, the synchronicity, the phone calls, and the choices that ultimately led to one of the best decisions of my life.

There is a big difference between honoring the ego-self and honoring the True Self. The ego-self is the separate self, the small-self. The ego-self always wants to get its way. Usually, it will be to the detriment of someone else. Do not let that hold you back from honoring the True Self. Honoring the True Self will never be to the detriment of another; in fact, it will always, always, benefit everyone else. Honoring the True Self will feel light, joyful, and freeing. It will resonate throughout all parts of you even if it pisses somebody off, even if it scares the mind into thinking you are going to lose something, even if it goes against the program and what the program says is the "right" thing to do.

Many people I have seen, especially those with autoimmune diseases, are living in obligation; they are doing what they think other people need them to do. They are doing what is expected. They are people-pleasing. They are saying *yes* even when it is a *no*, and it is always depleting to them. A woman I treated had severe MS. Her body was breaking down, she was becoming weak, she could no longer walk, and she was using a walker and a wheelchair.

Through the work of developing inner connection, she realized she had lived her whole life in obligation. She was taking care of her sick mother, and she never said no to her needy neighbor nor to her sister who always had problems. She thought being a good person meant serving everyone else. Certainly, when you are in the True Self you are always in service to others because honoring the True Self is going to benefit everyone. But from the small-self and obligation, giving and giving to everyone else is always going to be depleting to you and to them.

Once she recognized this pattern and made a choice to honor what was true for herself unconditionally, she began to get her health back. She said no when it was truly a *no*. She made new arrangements with people, letting them know she could not continue to do these services for them anymore because it was not true for her; it was not truly feeding her, not working out for her. She let go of some relationships. She changed the relationship with her sister. Instead of always being a sounding board, she let her sister know it did not feel good for her and suggested they have a different arrangement where there could be something higher and more possible for both of them.

Some of the people she made rearrangements with were upset and tried to make her wrong and put her down. It was okay, though, because she was clear on what was right. She realized had it been a year earlier before we did this work together, she would have succumbed to the guilt; she would have felt terrible about herself and immediately run back into the old arrangements and agreements.

She held her ground because she knew feeding and nurturing her body were more important than taking care of everybody else's needs. Her real friendships were strengthened. People came around and told her, "I am so sorry I ever treated you the way I did. I don't want it to be like that. Let's have a new relationship." Even her sister, who at first was upset and withdrew, came back around into a new relationship that honored both of them. Her life sorted itself out when she made choices to honor her *Self.* The illness resolved, and she regained her health and the ability to walk.

When we drop into the True Self and listen to the heart, honoring what makes us come alive, it nurtures our body.

Even "life-threatening" diseases, illnesses we're told will not go away and will continue to get worse, are only persistent if we continue to hold ourselves in the old consciousness, in the old electromagnetic communication.

When we make a change at the root level everything changes. This is why a dis-ease like MS can resolve. Had she continued in the old patterns and old consciousness, being the old self, the disease would have progressed. Yes, the doctors are right about that. They typically are simply not aware that much can be done to shift that. When you do, all bets are off. It's a whole new scenario. You always have the choice to change who you think you are and align with the Self.

I worked with an amazing woman who had been diagnosed with Ehlers-Danlos Syndrome, a genetic disease involving the connective tissue, who had the same kind of turnaround. She also was in a wheelchair; she was at the chiropractor at least three times a week due to excruciating pain when her joints would sublux and easily come out of alignment. Ehlers-Danlos is where the connective tissue is stretchier than it should be, so it does not have the full integrity to hold the bony structure together.

Her hip or sacrum would frequently dislocate, so she could not walk around without dislocating her body. Her life revolved around her illness, and she saw a dire future.

When I evaluated her, it was clear she was in a faulty alignment at her foundation. When I looked at why her spine kept coming out of alignment, I could see the instability was coming from the bottom up. She had no foundation of security within herself. She was trying to be what everyone else wanted her to be. She had energetically left her own center and was defining herself based on who she was to everyone else. There are many reasons our system will do this. Many of us have had childhood experiences that instilled a sense our value and worth—and therefore survival—are secure when others are happy with us. Our subconscious, therefore, sets it up so we're always fulfilling others' needs. The information our nervous system pays attention to—again, usually unconsciously—and behaviors are all in place to secure our survival. In fact, they're destroying it.

This woman was standing on an unstable foundation and had no sense of her own center. Of course her sacrum couldn't stay in place.

After doing this work, she established a new inner alignment grounded in her own integrity from the foundation up, from the sacrum up. This was a solid, strong, unshakable sense of Self. When she made this foundational shift, her sacrum came back into ideal alignment. I could see the strength in this, and her body had the integrity to hold itself together. Her hips no longer dislocated, and she got out of the wheelchair. She began walking, homeschooling her child, doing work she loves, and living a meaningful life. She shared all of this with our community. A year later, she reached out to me again and said, "I never imagined my life could have expanded like this. My relationships, my work, and my relationship with my children have gotten better and better. As I have honored myself, that alignment has expanded into everyone around me, and I am seeing my life and world flourish." Her life continues to expand year by year in ways she never would have imagined possible.

It's a powerful story because in medicine we tend to think genetic diseases are not amenable to this type of work. When there is something physical or structural in the body, many think the inner workings of the mind have no jurisdiction over that. However, everything in us is listening to our inner dialogue. All of it is influenced. All of it can be changed.

When we come into our true integrity and alignment, and we honor that, it changes our genetics and connective tissue. Instead of expression of disease, we live in expression of health. Her former self never would have made this choice. She was in too much guilt over not doing what everyone else wanted. She was taught that. That is the small-self serving itself. It was not serving anyone for her to diminish and compromise herself.

Don't be afraid if you have held this pattern of putting everyone else first. This is not about selfishness. When we honor the Self, the True Self, everybody benefits. We are connected. We are not separate. When we live in the alignment of the true Self with a capital S, we know who we are. We do not live the lie, the projection, the fabrication, of the program—like a robot. We live as the True Self. Because the body is alive and is electromagnetic, when it is expressing alignment, we light up like a Christmas tree. We become a vibrant electromagnetic energy field moving across the planet allowing and inviting the illumination of everyone around us.

Let Others Not Like You

When we honor our True Self, it is going to be inconvenient for those with whom we have made unconscious agreements. We may have unconsciously agreed to cater to their needs above our own or to enable them to walk all over us without protest. Although deep inside, no one would consciously choose to give their power away or be in this kind of exchange, many of us are not aware we are doing this. We don't know we have infinite power within and do not need to compromise. I've seen so many people—myself included—making subconscious agreements to keep giving our power away out of guilt or a sense of needing to prove ourselves. We will always find others who will take it. It's okay to see these patterns and make a new choice.

When you rearrange and honor yourself, others may guilt you and make you wrong. They may throw insults at you; they may tell people bad things about you. If you are identified with the small-self and the program, this will sting. It may feel intolerable. The small-self needs to protect itself and will try to get your attention and get you to put your energy into fighting this. Don't let it. If you remember: *Life is happening for me*, and you invite the experience, you let that experience show you exactly where those lies live in your body.

Is there a pressure in your chest? Is there a heaviness in your belly? Is there a speeding up of urgency in your throat and you just have to prove to them they're wrong about you?

That is where those programs got lodged into your system. That is all that is; it is an experience showing you what you are ready to let go of. When you do, the external situation will change. Manipulative people will either fall away from your life, or they will shift and no longer have the ability to abuse or control you.

Are you willing to invite and breathe that guilt rather than continue to self-medicate by complying with the co-dependent relationships?

For you to live freely, you must let other people have their pain and have their judgment about you. You must be willing to breathe through the experience and let it go. As soon as you do this, you are no longer holding judgment against yourself, so it does not matter if someone judges you. It does not matter if someone hates you or throws insults at you. There will be no hooks in you for them to grab onto. You can let them have their experience and those ideas about you and stay perfectly at peace because *you no longer believe those things to be true about yourself.* Any time you are triggered by another who wants you to stay in the old alignment, who wants you to keep compromising yourself to do what they want you to do, it is an experience to show you where you bought into a lie. It is arising because you are now ready to let go of that lie so *you* can live more freely.

Anytime this comes up, see the energy of that person going back to them. You do not need to carry their energy. You do not need to reconcile their energy. You do not need to school them in any way because you are giving them their energy back. *The only place their energy can resolve is within them.*

Giving someone back their pain is one of the most loving and compassionate acts you can do.

For most people, until they feel their pain, they will not be willing to change their behavior. They will not be willing to change who they are. They will not even see what's really causing their problem.

I've seen this often with parents. So many clients have told me, "My adult child isn't talking to me. I don't know what I did. I just want to love them, and they won't even see me." Or, "My child is cruel to me; I'm only trying to help them."

We don't see we've been parenting from control, trying to do it for them, holding onto our kids' energy. We don't see where we're parenting from fear. We don't want them to have pain. I've seen dozens and dozens practice this work and witness a miraculous turnaround. One of the greatest gifts you can give someone is their own pain. You are letting go of their energy and letting them have it. You are letting the energy work itself out in the only space it can: within themselves. Our experiences grow us; it's resisting our experiences that kill us. It's a profound gesture of courage, especially as a parent, because we think we're supposed to help our child avoid pain. Trust that your child or loved one has just as much connection to Source as you do, and that when met with their own pain, they can also make the choice to surrender.

> *The most precious gift we can offer others is our presence.*
> ~ Thich Nhat Hanh

It can be uncomfortable to watch someone suffer, but remember: They are already whole, just as you are. They are just as connected to Source as you are, not any more or less. You can only truly *love* them from compassion and from wholeness instead of loving them from your brokenness and fear, seeing them, too, as broken. What if that person is as capable of awakening as you are, and you give them back their pain instead of trying to take it on yourself?

You are empowering them to have their own awakening and to regain their own power. Sometimes it takes a lot of courage. Courage is of the heart. Courage is a form of love. It activates the electromagnetics of your heart and keeps you in your strongest alignment. You need to have courage in order to walk this path. It can be scary, especially when your whole foundation of community or resources is dependent on other people liking you. If you let them go, you think you are going to let go of money or love or belonging.

Remember, that person is not your source. Your job is not your source. Your family is not your source. Your husband is not your source. *Source* is your source. When you reconnect with Source as your source, you will always be provided for. You will always be strengthened. You will always be in your clarity, and you will always be in your peace. Letting people go can create a temporary appearance of loss. Some people may reject you, and it may seem you are letting go of the most important things in your life. But I guarantee, if you continue to hold your true inner alignment, true resources will come. True strength will come. True belonging will come, and your life will rearrange around your Truth.

EVERYTHING IS HAPPENING FOR YOU— RECEIVE INSTEAD OF RESIST

Can you see how everything shared here is pointing you to the truth that the Universe is on your side?

Everything taking place in your life is serving your highest alignment with Truth; it is serving your awakening. When you realize this, you partner with life. Instead of resisting it or fearing it or trying to make it different, you get into alignment with it because you realize it is cultivating your courage, strength, integrity, and healing. Once you realize this, it is a lot easier to release resistance and embrace what is happening in your life instead of fearing it. This can be challenging when there are diseases or severe symptoms in your body. But if you let in some of these principles and find the courage to soften your body, you are going to realize this is true, and everything is serving you.

Now you realize you have a choice. You can clamp down, tense up, and white-knuckle your way through life, trying to use your power and your strength to get what you want to manifest health. Or you can open. You can soften. You can receive life, and you can let this infinite resource here on your behalf come through you to manifest it all for you.

It is important to ask yourself: *Am I open and receptive, or am I in closure?*

Developing moment-to-moment awareness serves you. If you begin to trust life is on your side and everything is happening for you, you can surrender and let go. In so doing, you receive the greatest health, wealth, and love. Now the question becomes: *Am I in receptivity or closure?* That awareness is key. You have lots of tools that will help you stay in openness, which allows more expansion. It is important to tune into awareness.

This is where the 3-Step Instant Elevation Technique comes in. I became aware of it when I began teaching this work, and many people asked me, "How do you heal yourself? How do you cultivate that power and clear away the old energy?"

I checked in and witnessed my process could be broken down into three steps. When we learn these steps, they become automated in our system. It happens on autopilot and keeps us vibrating at a higher frequency. It works instantly to let our system release the old programs and immediately align with Truth.

Instant Elevation, introduced in Chapter Two, is a way to develop more awareness of your vibrational frequency, starting with the physical body.

The first step is to cultivate that awareness and strengthen your ability to be fully here, now. You may not be aware of your emotions; you may not be aware of what's going on mentally, but you *can* become aware of the sensations you are having in your body right now. This is a portal to power.

The body lives only in the now. It cannot live in the future. It cannot live in the past. It cannot live in the small-self identity, which is a projection of who you think you are supposed to be. It can only live in the now. So get yourself here now. Bring your attention to the physical sensations you are having right now, soften your shoulders and take a few breaths, and this will shift your brain.

You are recalibrating your nervous system and your electromagnetic system, your frequency. Even if you are in closure and you are white-knuckling it and clamping down in a ton of fear—having the *awareness* you are clamping down in fear is a higher frequency state, and it will shift what is happening. Developing the ability to tune into this awareness is the first step of your practice and the most essential one.

So, notice: *Am I receptive or am I in closure?*

Forgive Yourself for Resisting Life, and Stop Making It Wrong

How do we leave resistance behind and return to receptivity? You want your life to flow—meaning your body is functioning more ideally, and your electromagnetics are more in harmony. One of the best ways to accomplish this is to stop making what is happening now *wrong*.

When I asked you a moment ago to drop into your body and allow in sensation, was there pain, was there tightness, was there discomfort?

What did you do with it?

Notice that. Then notice what you made it mean. When I was sick with an "autoimmune disorder" I fell into a lot of fear every time I felt my back go into spasm, felt my neck pain, or felt overwhelmed with my fatigue. I made what was happening to me wrong. I would think: *Why is this happening? Nothing is working. I have to fix it. I have to fight this.*

Once I developed awareness, I could recognize what I was doing. I was fighting and clamping down against the sensations in my body. If I allowed the sensation or let my body know it was okay to feel what I was feeling and let go, my body would soften, and the pain would immediately go away. There were no more spasms or back pain. Even if it came back later, I would practice again and again. Eventually, the whole pattern would resolve completely. I made the choice to stop fearing those sensations, to stop fearing those experiences and to let them in.

The pain was just energy moving through. It was there to show me something. It was reflecting the tension I was holding. If I could be soft with myself, I would begin to see. If I stayed receptive and let go, my body could heal.

To be truly free, we must feel our emotions with full acceptance.
Then they quickly dissolve, because embracing and
fully accepting them is an act of unconditional love,
and darkness dissolves in the light of love.
~ Ziad Masri, *Reality Unveiled*

Sometimes you may embrace what's arising in the moment, and the pain does not go away immediately. You just develop awareness. Just let that in. You witness the process you are in, your relationship with pain, and let it continue to show you what this part of you needs. Forgive that it is happening. Forgive yourself. Forgive the illness. Forgive the experience and stop making it wrong. That is the most essential choice you can make once you start having awareness about what is going on within you—once you start having the awareness you are in closure.

Release the need for this to be instant. Attachment will only hinder the process. One of my greatest osteopathic mentors, Dr. Donald Hankinson, told me "When you approach your patient like you have all day, it will take five minutes. When you approach your patient like you have five minutes, it will take all day."

The same is true for your body. It will feel your attachment, which is closure, and it will respond accordingly. Stay open to however the process unfolds for you. Keep the intention to be well, but surrender your attachment.

You Open, and Life Does the Work

With everything I had learned about MindBody Medicine and self-healing, I somehow thought healing was supposed to come *from* me—like I was supposed to get smart enough or strong enough to do something different and make my body get better and stronger. This was the very thing keeping me sick because it was such a stress state to be taking on. Instead, I learned by no longer making the sensations, fatigue, and illness *wrong*, I could let go. More energy and compassion would course through me. That allowed the pain and illness to resolve. My energy came back, and the fatigue resolved as I allowed this surrender within.

I did not *create* the life force that came in and healed my body. I opened to allow more of it to course through me. It was dramatic to witness my body heal. Within days, pain and fatigue stopped coming back. I stopped having to remind myself over and over to shift my focus, to embrace and love myself, to physically soften my body. These became automatic functions in my system. I walked around feeling and being softer. I walked around with more self-acceptance. I walked around in more compassion, so my body functioned at a higher level.

The most important thing I released was trying to heal myself, which had created just another stress state. It was my small-self ego's to-do list, trying to escape failure, manage my life, heal my body, and do all the *right* things. It was a program.

Doing all of this in the belief I had to heal myself was only feeding the ego, and the ego is the one who was carrying the illness programs.

When we remember: *I can open,* and *life moves through me,* we leave the heavy lifting to the Universe. You did not create your liver, kidneys, and blood cells. You do not have to repair them either. But you *can* soften and allow receptivity so the Life Force that created you and is still moving through you can course through to a much higher degree. When you choose to receive instead of resist life, you come into alignment with that Life Force. You open to let more of it course through you for the creation of a healthy body and a vibrant, miraculous, powerful life of great joy and contribution.

Now that you have begun to cultivate deeper courage and compassion, you can open in the deepest spaces within you. This is when you are ready to begin receiving far more in life. In the next chapter, I walk you through how to open even more fully, into the deepest spaces, so that you become the ultimate receiver. This expansion in your ability to receive life greatly ignites the power within you for instant healing.

CHAPTER FIVE

Let Your Biggest Problem Be Your Greatest Gift

What if you were to stop seeing your problem or illness as a punishment, or even as a negative thing, and start relating to it as pure energy?

What if you were to stop making it wrong, fighting against it, trying to solve it, trying to make it go away—and instead, were willing to receive the moment exactly as it is?

Would there be more peace in your moment right now, would your shoulders be more relaxed, would you be breathing more fully, knowing there is nothing you have to do?

As soon as you let go of the fight that creates so much stress and resistance in your system, you enter a new dimension of consciousness. It may look like everything is the same, and everything may feel like it is the same, but as soon as you shift—even micro-shift—in your perspective from: *I have to solve this problem* to *I can accept this moment exactly as it is*, you shift everything.

What if this moment, exactly as it is, is a gift and is serving you?

What if something about this experience is growing you in some essential and important way?

You shift your consciousness. That micro-shift in consciousness makes all the difference in what is happening cellularly.

A young client named River recently came to me with severe, unrelenting pain. She had been to multiple physicians and specialists for pain, pediatric neurology, pediatric orthopedics, and sports medicine, to no avail. She had been doing physical therapy for months, but the pain was only becoming worse. She was diagnosed with RSD, Reflex Sympathetic Dystrophy, and she was put on strong pain medications. Despite continued treatment by various doctors, River had been debilitated for months, sleeping on the couch in the living room and unable to climb the stairs to her bedroom or to bathe. Her mother had been washing her hair in the living room, catering to her every need including toileting, and had witnessed her own life become consumed with caring for her daughter.

Multiple times, an ambulance had been called to the house to get River off the floor and bring her to the hospital because the symptoms were so severe, she was writhing in pain and screaming. She had been admitted several times to the hospital for pain management and more diagnostic testing. Her parents were at their wits' end. Finally, River was ready to see me to try a new approach. We set up a brief session over Zoom.

I explained to River that sometimes our unconscious tries to get our needs met in ways we've been unable to meet ourselves, even if they didn't make sense. When I asked her to list any ways she could possibly imagine that this illness might be serving some of her needs, she was willing to be open-minded and consider this.

She then shared, "I really didn't want to go to school, and now I don't have to." And "I've been able to relax and do things in my own time; I don't have to rush or be busy anymore." There were a few other items she listed, and I could feel her system lightening up. There was still a nugget there though.

"Is there anything else you can think of that this illness is serving, perhaps trying to take care of something for you?"

Immediately she lit up. "My sister isn't mean to me anymore. She's nice and we have a good relationship."

I witnessed an immense amount of energy release from her system like she'd had a big exhale. "Tell me more," I said.

It turns out her older sister would be very hard on her when her friends were over playing games and sports. Young River was very empathic and would try to toughen up, not letting her emotions be apparent, not letting her sister know this hurt her, and trying to be tough.

There it was. I could feel the "Trying to be tough and suppress my emotions" pattern playing. She had learned this through these interactions, and this was extremely detrimental to her system. River is here to be empathic and sensitive, and if this were to be turned off, it was clear she would not meet her life's purpose.

"*Aha!* We've got it!" I said. "Do you see how toughening up is not serving you? Do you know it's okay to share your feelings and let others see when something hurts you? Your sister loves you but what works for her is not necessarily what works for you," I said. "Are you ready to stay sensitive and let people see how things make you feel, so you can ask for what you need, and they can adjust their behavior?

River was absolutely on board for this, being the empathic and very intelligent youngster she was. We did some EFT (Emotional Freedom Technique) Tapping to move anything related to this out of her system and bring in the strength and knowing that being sensitive was a superpower, and she could trust it.

That very evening, River climbed the stairs and slept in her own bed. The next morning, she bathed and was able to walk outside. Within days, she was ready to go back to school and rejoin her team for volleyball.

This is how quickly things can shift when we are willing to let in the experience and receive the gift it has for us.

I invite you to ask yourself: *Is there anything good about this?*

This can be difficult to see, especially if you are in a serious hardship, facing something that is life-threatening, or you are in debilitating pain. This is not about trying to have a "putting-ice-cream-on-top-of-poop positive thinking mindset." Finding the gift is not about glossing over what is happening. We are going deep down into the pain to witness what is there. This is what allows the breath and the light to come in at that level. This allows you to make the true, solid, and profound shift in your consciousness so there is a true and solid shift in everything happening physically. The most productive way to do that is to stop approaching the illness as a problem and get curious about how your current circumstances could be serving you.

YOU HEAL WHEN YOU STOP BEING THE FALSE YOU

Your body is your greatest feedback device. If you let go of seeing it as a solid physical object and see it instead as a vessel through which you can awaken, you let in the possibilities that your vessel, your body, is trying to show you. Most of us are playing the game of life unconsciously. We use our bodies like a chess piece or an avatar and become completely identified with it, forgetting who we are. It's like when you are in a video game and you get set up with an image of a little person who looks like you. You give it your hair color or the hair color you think is fun. You choose its clothing. You make it look how you want to appear in the video game. It's the same on social media—you choose a favorite picture of yourself as a profile, and that picture represents you.

Every time you make a comment, is the little picture making the comment? Of course not. *You* are making the comment, and the picture image is representing you. Do you lose sight of the fact the image or avatar is not actually *you?* It is easy to understand how this could happen when we become really involved in the virtual world or are playing a video game. We become attached to what's happening in the game. When our avatar fails, we feel it. When our avatar dies, we're bummed.

Imagine now getting even more involved. Imagine being so into the game, you forget it's just a game. You become so attached to the outcome, it dictates how you feel moment to moment. You no longer have peace. You feel good only when the avatar is winning, and you feel bad when the avatar is not.

Now imagine being so involved in that reality, you forget who you are and start believing you *are* the avatar. Everything the avatar experiences, you experience. If the avatar is abandoned by a lover, you suffer. If the avatar loses money, you feel anger and loss. If the game piece is slandered, you feel shame. If the game piece dies, you die. This is what is happening with the body. The real you—the *I AM* that you truly are—is not your body. If you are identified with the body, it seems like the body is you, it is who you are, and you become very identified with what you look like, how you feel, what kind of status you have in this reality, and what kind of image other people have of you. Your identity or how you feel, who you think you are gets all tied up and vested in those factors outside you. None of those factors are the True Self.

What if you remember your body is really your feedback device to show you when you are out of alignment with the truth? What if the truth is simply that I AM—*I*, being the consciousness of All That Is and *AM* being the embodiment of All That Is. The existence of All That Is. What if the whole purpose of what you are doing here in this realm we call "reality" is to awaken to that truth? Everywhere you are out of alignment, you are overly identifying with your status—or other peoples' ideas about you or your physical looks, or the status of your physical body—and it is going to bring discord. It is going to bring resistance to your system, and your body is simply going to let you know about that. Your body says to you: *You have come out of alignment with the I AM, with the presence of All That Is, with the alignment of eternal flow. Heads up!*

Some people call that eternal presence *God*. Some people call it *Spirit*. Some people call it *The Universe*. You might call it *Divine Presence*. I sometimes call it the *Innate Intelligence*. But what you call it is not what's important. What matters is whether you are allowing an authentic connection with this presence of Oneness Consciousness. This is the truth of the I AM. This is the truth of what you truly are, and your embodiment can be a reflection of that instead of reflecting the limited small-self. When you are in alignment with the Divine flow and with the power and majesty of who you are, your body receives that. You are open to receiving the Divine Intelligence and the Divine Intelligence is feeding and fueling your body and your self.

When you are out of alignment with your true nature, the opposite happens. The body is in discord; there is resistance. Energy cannot move and there is pain. Maybe there is inflammation, so disease develops and you get a diagnosis. The point is not that the diagnosis is the reality; the point is your body is showing you where you bought into a faulty conclusion and you closed. It's showing you where you are out of alignment with your Truth. That is the false you.

If you are awakening into the True You, then what is the false you?

The false you is simply all of your old ideas, conclusions, and beliefs that got instilled from all the unresolved pains, hurts, abandonment, or traumas you have experienced and caused you to shut down. This false you is holding tension. You are afraid. You are sure life is not on your side and you cannot let go of control. You have bought into the conclusion that you are not safe, so you hold yourself in a certain amount of restriction and limitation.

That is going to set up the system for what is happening in your adrenal glands, kidneys, digestive and reproductive organs, metabolism, and even your DNA. Every part of your system is either under the program of that false-self, holding and resisting and fighting, which is generating inflammation and disease, or it is under the guidance of True Self, which is the space of wholeness, health, purity, flow, and perfection.

If you were to realize your body is your feedback device, and it is on your side for your well-being, would you be more open and surrendered?

Would you be more willing to soften and allow this moment to be as it is?

I know there may be pain, and I know there may be severe fatigue and unthinkable discomfort or fear in any given moment, but consider that your softening and breathing more deeply lets that energy move so it does not stay stuck in your physical body.

When you receive the Truth your body is your feedback device, assisting your awakening, it immediately shifts your relationship with your body. This shifts your brain activity. It shifts your chemistry and your hormones, and it very importantly shifts your electromagnetic field.

The electromagnetic field is the most potent, most primary determinant of what is happening in your body, the quality of your health, and the quality of your experiences.

Are you in an energy field where possibilities exist, where there is ease and flow, where things turn out for you, where things happen fluidly, and where life works out easily for you? Or are you in an electromagnetic field where no matter what you do, there is always more you have to deal with, or where you have to keep working hard and it never quite works out for you?

Usually when we are facing a mountain that is circumstantial, we are facing the reality of life. When we are facing a mountain that is chronic, we are facing a reality of ourselves.
~ Brianna West, *The Mountain Is You*

The other day, I heard my husband telling his friend about a vacation we had in Santa Fe. He was explaining we had booked a special resort away from the town center where we usually stay, because it had a nice pool and hot tub and great space for the kids. A week before we checked in, we got an email from the resort letting us know all of the pool facilities were under renovation. Our big plan had fallen apart.

Then I overheard his friend sarcastically say, "Of course, isn't that always how things go? Just when you try to make it good, things always fall apart."

That is the response many people would have. There's this idea that life is always going to let you down when you least expect it, and the other shoe is going to drop. It's true when you keep seeing it that way.

But, is that True? You have to realize life is almost always working out exactly the way we want it. Life is always on our side. Catch yourself in those moments when you buy into the idea: *Of course this happens to me,* and choose not speak that way anymore because your words are power; your words are creative.

Are there aspects in your reality you decide are bad and unwanted, so you affirm Life is against you?

Start breaking that habit right now. Notice when you are doing that and pause. Ask yourself: *What if this is to my benefit?* We ended up having a super fun time with the kids playing around in the room. They created new games together and a lot of cool memories came out of the vacation. We didn't swim, and it didn't matter. If I can receive the experience instead of rejecting it, I am in a better place.

When you do this, you are in greater flow; you are allowing more of the intelligent Life Force to flow through your body and your mind, to flow into your life and create miraculous circumstances for you.

Closure Creates Disease

Your body physicalizes the energy and consciousness in which you function. Your body amplifies the energy so you can notice. Usually this is unconscious. Most of us are not aware of the frequency we are functioning in, which is fine because the body brings the awareness to us.

If you are an energy-sensitive or empathic or highly sensitive person (HSP), and you are dialed into energy, you may feel right away when something happens that puts you in a lower frequency. Maybe someone says something that triggers you and makes you feel bad or brings up an old wound or causes you to feel powerless and threatened. You immediately feel: *I am taking on this person's energy.*

This is great because you can nip it in the bud. You have the ability to pause, remember to soften your body, and let that energy dissipate. The breath can let that energy release. The awareness can let that energy release. Then it doesn't get stuck in the body and create dis-ease, illness, and pain. It doesn't hang out in the body and affect your electromagnetic field and cause more drama and trauma in your life.

However, let's say you are not so energy-sensitive. Maybe you are more identified with the physical level, and this idea about underlying energy is all very new to you. It does not matter because the body is going to give you feedback at whatever level you are paying attention. Many people are disconnected and not tuned into the energy body or aware of their emotions. They're not aware of what they are feeling inside and are only aware of the physical. Even that may be numbed with distractions, addictions, recreational drugs, or medications. Sometimes people want to disconnect from all sensation. It's okay. Your body is going to keep screaming louder, trying to bring your attention back to the now, back into your feedback system. Perhaps a disease requiring medications comes along and just won't go away, and it's time for you to look deeper at what's happening.

Your body is your partner in your awakening process. It's going to do everything to bring up repressed emotions, so you can make a new choice and finally release them. If the energy is suppressed at the emotional level, it will certainly present itself at the physical level. The energy has to move.

A good friend of mine developed severe chest pain and shortness of breath. He went to the hospital repeatedly but was told nothing was wrong. My friend was familiar with my work and knew her brother harbored lots of unresolved emotions around their father's recent death. He'd never dealt with the issues in their relationship or his feelings of loss. He didn't express sadness or talk about their dad's death. She was aware there were likely repressed emotions at the root of this recurrent severe chest pain and encouraged him to reach out to me. Her brother eventually called me for some help because no one else could help him with the chest pain, and he had now developed severe anxiety. He couldn't figure out what was going on. I pointed out grief can do this and the symptoms were likely related to the loss of his father.

"It's not that," he said. "I'm not upset about my dad dying. I mean, it's sad, but I'm not even thinking about it."

"Exactly," I said. "You've suppressed the emotions, so the energy is coming up physically." We did some EFT Tapping, and he was able to experience a resolution.

What we repress emotionally will eventually resurface as physical symptoms. The energy has to go somewhere. When it's repressed, it disrupts the physical body, and we feel it. In fact, when someone comes to me with chronic physical pain, most often they are not aware at all of the underlying emotions. They'll protest over and over, telling me, "This is physical. There's nothing emotional going on."

And that's exactly the point. If they were aware of their emotions, the energy would move, and it wouldn't be creating the physical symptoms. Not being conscious of the emotions doesn't mean they're not there. Few people are fully aware of all the emotional energy they're carrying. It's typically a matter of time until it manifests on the physical level so it can be dealt with.

This can happen when life triggers us into an upset. Let's say someone hits your car. It's a minor incident, but if you're harboring repressed emotions, it makes you feel angry. Maybe you think: *Now I am going to have thousands of dollars in damage. Life is always trying to get me.* Maybe you've just made a choice to decrease your job to part-time to have more ease and abundance in your life. However, if you have not increased your consciousness of money and abundance, the events seem threatening. You think: *Now I'm really in trouble. I shouldn't have let go of my full-time job. Life's out to get me, and I can't win.*

What will you do the next time circumstances seem to be threatening?

Will you buy into the old thoughts and clamp down into control and tension?

There's a choice. The experiences will bring up energies that already live within you, and they give you the opportunity to let them go so you move into greater expansion. Take it.

If triggers arise, you can tune in and be present in your body. You will feel the heaviness, anger, or fear that may be there. Maybe you feel a twist in your stomach, a pressure on your shoulders, or heaviness in your chest. You can soften your body and tune into the experience at a deeper level. The energy will release. As you breathe, you exhale the emotional energy the incident brings up for you.

Maybe you do not feel any emotions and you fight against the experience. You tense your body and try to figure out how to make things work, or you call your employer and beg to go back to full-time—anything to go back to your comfort zone.

You're too scared to honor your previous choice now that you've been challenged. You go back to the baseline tension of anger or fear your system has become accustomed to. You push down the emotions that arise and vow never to listen to your heart again. For a while, it may seem that all is well, but the energy has to go somewhere. Eventually, physical symptoms arise—pain in your shoulders, indigestion, headaches. It's going to keep giving you the opportunity to choose in favor of your expansion.

When you remain in closure, the energy gets pushed farther downstream. The nervous system remains in fight-or-flight, inflammation continues, and this will likely develop into overt illness. Maybe you get a diagnosis of inflammatory bowel syndrome or autoimmune disease. The body will physically manifest the energy you have suppressed.

If you're not aware of the underlying thoughts, emotions, sensations, and energy, it will seem like it came out of nowhere. You'll be dumbfounded about why this happened to you, or worse, you'll make it into a story that life is against you, bringing you one bad thing after another. Life is trying to get your attention at the level where you are paying attention. What you do with that experience is up to you.

Life can get your attention upstream, when the trigger first happens and you feel the subtle energies—or downstream, after you've repressed those more subtle levels and things begin to manifest on more of a physical level. It does not matter at which point the system gets your attention. It matters what you do when it does. In the early stage, soften your body, take a few deep breaths, and let that energy move. Immediately you align with Life and come into the moment. When you do, you are provided with everything you need—money to pay for the car, resources to take care of things, and the energy, insight, and ideas that make life sort out smoothly. The resources are included in the package. Maybe you even make a friend in a car collision and have an exchange of kindness and compassion, which I, myself, have experienced.

You can tune in at whatever point you are along the trajectory. Maybe you feel the fear and immediately tell yourself: *Body, it is okay, you can let go of this fear. Let go of those ideas about lack. We will receive exactly what we need.* You do a rewrite and rectify the energy in the present moment before it stews and percolates into something more physical. Maybe you are totally unaware of what is happening and it's not until further downstream, maybe ten years of stewing in fear and lack and frustration about life not going your way—and you get a medical diagnosis. In that moment you can do the same thing. You can receive it and ask: *What will this illness show me if I am willing to receive it?*

You do not have to answer the question of *Why is this happening?* or *What is going on here?* or *What is the message?* because the mind cannot compute that when you are in lower consciousness. But if you simply pause the moment a pain comes up or something triggers you—such as receiving a diagnosis—relax your body and ask: *What would it take for me to receive this with grace and ease and allow everything to change?*

This is the moment that can change your life. The miracle is that your body is not going to quit on you. It is not going to just manifest that low-frequency energy. It will keep trying to get your attention so you can make a change.

Maybe the message is being reflected in your relationships, and you've had, as I did, relationship disaster after relationship disaster. Maybe you are always in financial misery and lack, struggling to make ends meet or always worried about money. Many of you reading this book may be asking: *Why do I have this medical problem that will not go away? Why am I always sick? Why can't I get my health back?*

If you are asking questions similar to these—pause. Receive what is happening and ask: *How can this be happening for me? Am I willing to receive the sensations, the awareness, and any communication that my own wisdom is trying to tell me through this experience?*

Life Shows the Sum Total of Resistance

For those who understand this approach and wonder:

What am I holding onto?

How can I let go?

Is it from a specific trauma?

Is it from a past life?

Is it from when I was three?

Did it happen in the womb?

How do I know what I need to let go?

We do not necessarily need to answer any of those questions because we only have to deal with what is here *now*. As soon as you drop into sensation and soften your body and breathe, you are going to feel everything that is here now. The awesome thing is everything you need in order allow the greatest healing is here, right now in this moment. You can feel into bodily sensations—such as tightness in your chest, heaviness on your shoulders, cramping in your belly, or a butterfly feeling in your solar plexus. Tune into that now, soften, and let it in. Sometimes emotions like fear or dread will come up. Become aware of those feelings, sensations, emotions, and ideas. All of them lead you to the core of what is behind the energy.

Your body exists only in this now moment. As soon as you drop in, feel, and sense what is here, it is going to show you what needs to be brought to your attention. You may be carrying trauma from decades ago that is active in this moment, creating limitations in your health, relationships, or your money. You can tap into that energy in your body right here, right now. Sense and feel what is here.

You can ask questions that will key you into what you are holding:

What would allow more freedom in my finances?

What would be the best way for me to allow powerful love in my relationship?

What would it take for me to live my highest level of freedom and health?

Then get receptive. Soften. Breathe slowly. Being receptive is the biggest step so many skip over. You must allow your body to enter the parasympathetic state so there is receptivity to the wisdom and answers you're looking for.

You may feel physical sensations or emotions or become aware of the thoughts and ideas that go with them. Let all of those be as they are and just breathe into them. Your body is carrying remnants of the pain-body, which is the sum of all of your emotional pain and distress. Victim identity, trauma from being abandoned, and everything you are holding from your past is all right here, right now.

> *Painful feelings are just energies asking for their emancipation.*
> ~ Sarah Blondin, *Heart Minded*

The small-self, the identity who thinks: *I am not good enough, I always have to work hard,* or *no one loves me,* will also be present. That self shows up in the form of physical sensations, feelings, emotions, or the thoughts and beliefs that come up in the moment. The good news is everything happening is always leading you to your greatest power, your greatest awakening, and the resolution of everything you are ready to resolve in your life right now.

It will seem like you have diseases.I In medicine, we look at the body as separate. Medical practitioners will say things like

"You have thyroid disease; you have adrenal fatigue; you have an autoimmune process going on." There are more and more terms created every year for all the different things going on in your body that we label "disease." But the reality is *one thing*. There is one thing happening and that is your state of BE-ing right now.

Years back, a colleague referred a patient to me. Colleen had been bed-bound for three years and had suffered with severe pain, anxiety, and incapacitating fatigue. She had been diagnosed with Lyme disease, autoimmune illness, anxiety and panic disorder, and chronic fatigue syndrome. She came to me after seeing many doctors and having had only minimal improvement using medications, diet strategies, intravenous infusion therapies, supplements, and many other approaches.

Upon working together, it was clear Colleen's system was in an almost continuous fight-or-flight state. We uncovered multiple emotional traumas as well as limiting beliefs about herself. Most of these had been unconscious. Colleen had pushed herself hard to overcome her illness, finish college, and try to have a functional life. She was a fighter, and her illness was giving her the opportunity to show that. She had learned to push herself, but prior to that she had learned to shut down her emotions and hide her feelings. Toughness became a way of being. Underneath it all, Colleen felt like a victim, as if life was working against her, and she had to put all her energy into fighting.

I introduced her to the MindBody approach and the work that is now my Embracing Health program. We used EFT Tapping and other MindBody tools to resolve the mental and emotional root causes of what was consuming so much of her energy. We allowed a shift in her consciousness beyond fear and victimhood into love, prosperity, and power. Colleen began to see results right away. Her energy came back, and she was able to enjoy more activities. Her pain began to resolve, and she had more and more periods of feeling well. Most importantly, she began to see where her thoughts and beliefs were impacting her body. She began to notice when she fell into the perspective of victimhood and hopelessness and learned to breathe that energy out of her body. Over time, she regained power through surrender, instead of fighting. She started sharing her feelings instead of repressing them. She let go of relationships that were not serving her and strengthened the ones that did serve her. Through devotion to her inner power, over time, Colleen completely resolved the Lyme disease, autoimmune disease, chronic fatigue syndrome, and all other symptoms.

Her doctors were dumbfounded.

Colleen did not need to figure out and solve all the separate illnesses, and neither do you. There is one foundational energy behind all of it, and that is *the electromagnetic frequency you are residing in right now.* That frequency or consciousness is the sum of all the hurts and all the tensions and all the resentments and all the wounds and protections and all the unresolved emotions that are part of your system.

You do not have to deal with all of these separately; you can tune in right here, right now and your system will show you exactly what is ready to move. That allows the resolution of a thousand things we perceive as *disease.* If you've had multiple separate symptoms or been given several diagnoses, do not be afraid. Do not make it a *thing* to handle. You can go into the now moment and connect with your power, the Intelligence that designed you, and allow it to take care of resolving all of your symptoms.

THE MYTH OF DISEASE

What is disease? It can be helpful from the medical perspective to categorize symptoms into clusters that go together so we can understand the process someone is in. If someone has severe headaches, visual changes, and weakness, we might think they have had a stroke. We make a diagnosis about what is causing that cluster of symptoms. This is helpful when we understand the clear-cut medical reasons and are able to treat them.

With so much chronic illness in the world, we cluster the symptoms and give a diagnosis even when we do not understand the cause, and we do not have a successful way to treat them. Because so many people are living in a low-frequency consciousness, the body is not getting the health it needs. It is like the body is breaking down in a hundred different ways simultaneously.

What we practitioners call *disease* does not necessarily have a lot of meaning medically. We do not really understand why you are having that cluster of symptoms and we do not necessarily understand what to do for you to help resolve those symptoms. When you get a diagnosis like fibromyalgia or chronic fatigue syndrome, there may be a cluster of symptoms that go together, and you say: *Oh good; I am so grateful someone has finally identified what is wrong with me. I have* _____ (fill in the blank with the syndrome). But it does not necessarily tell us anything about why you have it or what to do about it.

Don't Give Your Diagnosis Too Much Power

People tend to give the diagnosis a power, an identity of its own. Then instead of a cluster of symptoms or a state their body is in right now, it becomes "*my* fibromyalgia," "*my* chronic fatigue," or "I have MS."

If you adopt this approach, you not only make it an entity that has an existence of its own, but you also make it *yours*, like it has taken over your body or it belongs to you; *it is who you are*. This is dangerous because as soon as you identify with a thing, you give it power, you give it its own life, you give it its own capability. The program of that disease, everything contained within that package, then exists and plays out in your system.

Most of these diseases or diagnoses have conclusions that go along with them. "If you have MS, it is going to get progressively worse, and you will have it for the rest of your life." "If you have cancer, there is nothing that can possibly be done besides chemotherapy." It is dangerous if you buy into those ideas because you begin to live them. You will not access other possibilities that could heal you, and the disease will continue to get worse if you continue to buy into it.

The disease itself is not an actual thing. It does not have a real life or an identity or real power. You have given a term to the state your body is in now. If you let go of the idea that the disease is a thing and has its own power, you no longer give it your life force and you stop creating that course.

From now on, instead of viewing what is happening to you as an illness or a disease, remember it is a state you are in right now; it is energy. See the energy of it in a new way. Allow the energy to move so it resolves here, now, and you no longer carry it with you.

Victim Consciousness: Life Is Happening *to* Me

Often when we have been given a disease diagnosis, we feel victimized. I witnessed this happening as soon as I got my diagnosis. I thought: *Oh no, I have this problem. I have this thing—this disease. I have to deal with this. I won't be okay.* I started thinking my life would never be the same. *I will never run again. I will never be pain-free and enjoy activity in my body.*

My doctor would have happily supported all of those conclusions and, in fact, did tell me I had to be on medication for the rest of my life. But none of those were true. I did not "have a thing." I realized I was in a state of inflammation. That inflammation was triggering my immune system. Then my immune system was responding in a very specific way that caused my lab work to look a certain way, and my symptoms felt a certain way that equaled "disease."

There was sensation, tension, and fear in my body. There was the *idea* I would never be okay or be able to truly live. I experienced sensations, emotions, thoughts, and ideas about what was happening.

I let go of the idea that something was happening to me and shifted out of victim consciousness. I asked: *How could this be happening for me? What is the gift here? What is my body trying to tell me?* and *How could this be the best thing that ever happened?* I instantly felt lighter and more relaxed.

That is exactly when I began to witness all the ways I had been fighting my body, battling through life trying to get ahead, trying to be better, and trying to avoid failure. I realized I had fear-of-failure programs running in my head. That was why my body was so clamped down, resistant, and tense. Those programs were generating the inflammation.

As soon as I released victim consciousness and realized Life is on my side and is happening for me, my body told me it was okay to let go. It told me: *You do not have to fight in life. You do not have to get somewhere. Life is on your side. You are already whole.* As soon as I embraced that, my whole body relaxed. It surrendered. It was a new cellular arrangement and my disease resolved within days.

Underneath the Illness

Instead of trying to battle a disease or your external circumstances, I invite you to enter the now moment and feel what is here.

Use Integration Exercise 3 from page 222 in this book and in your book bonuses at DrKimD.com/BYOHBonuses.

Even if you only do this for five minutes a day, you are going to move a lot more energy than you would otherwise move over ten or twenty years. Feel what is here. Breathe into your body and sense your breathing. Put your hand on your heart and focus attention there. Breathe slowly, relax your shoulders, and let them soften. The more you physically soften, the more sensation you allow.

The first thing you may notice is the idea: *I don't feel anything. I think I am doing it wrong.* That is fear, trying to protect you from having an experience. Instead of reacting to those thoughts and trying to *do it right*, let those thoughts in and welcome them because they are only natural. Other thoughts that may arise are: *I am broken; it's not working. I have been shut down too long. I will never feel anything. This will not apply to me.*

If you have been shut down for a long time, the brain will not immediately register a lot of sensation. But your brain is neuroplastic, meaning it has the ability to create new neural pathways and reform old ones, and it can pay attention to information in a new way. The body is already registering sensation, but you have not been paying attention to it, so it may not be readily apparent. Stay with the process. Drop in and feel your body. Sense your body. Bring your hand to your chest. Feel your breathing. Soften your shoulders and check in. Gently say: *Hi body. How are you?* Tune into what is here now. Is there a physical sensation, an emotion? Is there a thought like: *This is not working for me?* Welcome all those sensations and thoughts.

If there is a physical sensation, get curious and bring your attention there. Let the breath come more fully into that exact area and ask: *What do you have for me?* Sometimes an aspect of your small-self is clamping down in fear. You may feel anger, which is trying to protect you from something deeper, such as fear or shame. Get curious and bring your attention to that area with your breath.

Instead of calling this current state *my illness*, let it just be there: *Here I am, feeling this. Here I am, noticing this sensation. Here I am, having this thought.* When you bring attention to any area of your body and soften, you let the energy in that area move more fully. This can be challenging if there is fear or if there is overwhelm from a severe amount of pain. Feelings of despair, dread, powerlessness—the idea nothing you do will ever make a difference—can be difficult energies to breathe through. Breathe through them anyway. It is energy. As soon as you let it move, it is no longer part of your system, and it is no longer creating your experience. Breathe and soften to let that area move. The energy moves out, it is no longer held in, and it no longer creates disease.

If we are willing to let go of our illness, then we have to be willing to let go of the attitude that brought about the illness, because disease is an expression of one's attitude and habitual way of looking at things.
~David Hawkins, *Healing and Recovery*

When I was sick and had severe pain, I would clamp down in fear every time the pain came back. When I realized what was happening and interacted with my body in a new way, I would tell my back: *It's okay. You can let this go. I love you. I love you. I love you.* And I would send love to that area in my back every time I felt the pain—over and over again, each time it would come up. Within a number of days, the whole syndrome quieted down. I no longer let it be evidence that what I'm doing is not working. I let it be evidence that a part of me needed more loving attention. I was willing to give it that love and that presence and that breath. All I did was let my attention, awareness, and loving presence penetrate deeper into those areas in my body.

Your body will show you exactly what is needed. It is your job to facilitate receiving what the body most deeply needs.

YOUR ILLNESS AWAKENS YOU TO YOUR TRUE SELF

What if you realized the whole point of your illness or challenging experience is to awaken you to the truth?

Are you living in the program of thinking: *I have to keep going, then I will get ahead, and after I get XYZ done, then I will feel better and be free?* That is conditional and is never happening now; the freedom is not happening now. Life is trying to invite you to an experience of being free, and you have that experience of freedom right here, right now.

The True Self already knows peace because it *is* peace. The True Self already knows freedom because it *is* freedom. The True Self already knows abundance because it *is* abundance.

Any time you are living in any program of *less than*, it is painful. Any time you are putting your energy into something *less than*, it creates tension and problems. Any time you buy into a belief you are less than whole, your body shows you where you are out of true alignment. This happens to bring you into the experience of your peace and wholeness—to bring you into the experience of your joy, vitality, and abundance.

Remember your *illness* is only here to show you where something in you is out of alignment, and you are now capable of resolving it. Living as your True Self is way better than you imagine.

Most clients come to me to make their pain go away, resolve a chronic illness, help them get their energy back, or get rid of their chronic fatigue. They do not realize what is really in store for them is *so* much better than that. It is so much better than shutting off the symptoms and returning to their previous way of living.

You are not reading this book to simply fix a problem and get on with your life. You are here for something *so much bigger*. You didn't show up here and invest yourself by practicing an integration exercise five times a day just to *manage the stuff*.

When something appears in your life and calls for so much of your attention, it is so you can shift the foundation of *who you are* to create a massive, profound, meaningful, and valuable shift in everything you ever thought was possible for you, in everything you ever thought you could experience. Whatever got you here, thank it. Even though it can be so challenging you wish you never began the journey, it is always, always more than worth it.

Make some quiet time and ask yourself: *If all of this were worth it, and a year from now I was so grateful I could not believe it, jumping up and down with gratitude for how my life has changed because I surrendered and let this experience in, because I allowed this new way of being with myself, how would my life need to be for me to say having gone through the experience was more than worth it?*

Now make your list. Brainstorm. Go big. Nothing is beyond your capacity to create.

You can share it in the MindBody Community on Facebook at DrKimD.com/connect because I would love to hear from you.

Then you can learn more about every single thing you wrote on that list and more of what is in store for you. That is how amazing and worth it your True Self is.

Living the Programs Means Doing Things That Make You Sick

When you live in your small-self, victim identity, or pain-body, you continue doing things that create more resistance, like staying in a job you hate because you believe nothing else is out there for you. Or thinking you are not good enough to do what you want, so you drudge through your day like everyone else seems to be doing. Or maybe you stay in a relationship that is not your ideal alignment because you feel guilty about hurting your partner if you leave them. You may think you are not good enough to find someone better.

The time comes when you're ready to go beyond those beliefs. Something exists for you that is your ideal job, your ideal relationship, and you're ready. At that point, staying in the relationship will become even more painful; that job will become even more excruciating and suffocating.

When a higher match becomes available, you will feel it as either inspiration or desperation. Start listening to that pain or that challenge as the indicator. There is something much higher available for you now. When you live through that program, that small-self always has you running on a hamster wheel and doing things that assure your lack and limitation. Everything you do when you are in the pain-body is going to be to your own detriment. It is up to you to receive the moment and let it awaken you to realize you do not need to keep operating that way. Get curious. Be open.

Accessing the True-Self

It is so helpful to develop awareness of whether you are in the pain-body or in the True-Self. At any given moment you can check in: *Hi body. How are you?* Then rate the way you feel on a scale of 1 to 10. Ten is: *I feel vibrant, alive, fulfilled, and clear.* One is: *Oh my gosh I feel so miserable I can barely stand it.* Your response is information. Registering the awareness of where you are on the scale shifts your consciousness and your frequency.

Set an alarm for five times a day and do this in place of your Daily Integration practice:

Integration Exercise 3: Using Awareness to Shift Your State

- Relax and slow and deepen your breath.

- Bring your awareness to your body and check in with your body like you are lovingly greeting a friend: *Hi body. How are you?*

- Put your hand on your heart, feel your breath, and relax your shoulders. Assess where in this moment, you reside on a scale of 1 to 10, 10 being the highest state of joy. The information is enough. You do not need to fix it; there is nothing to fix. *The awareness is the medicine.*

- Welcome what you feel, whatever the number is. You can say: *It's okay I'm at a 5. I welcome the 5.* Welcome the energy of it into your heart.

- Send love to this part of you, to the one who is at a 5 or wherever you are. Say: *I love you.*

When you are in the True Self, you feel lightness, you feel purpose, you feel acceleration and fulfillment.

When you are operating on some level of the small-self, you are going to be aware of that. You may feel tension, pain, heaviness, or self-doubt. That is useful awareness to have.

Whenever you realize you are operating in anything lower than the True Self, welcome it and send yourself love.

Send love to the pain in your body. Send love to the one who is in fear. Send love to the one who is so sure they could never possibly make it and have a fulfilling life, who thinks that it will never work out for them. Send that one love. These are aspects of the self coming up to be healed.

And guess what heals them?

The power of your loving presence. That is it. That lets the breath come fully into the pain-body space so the energy can move and release those old hurts, pains, feelings of abandonment, and tensions. They are resolved from your system and are no longer there.

It is okay if you are at a 2, for instance. Do not judge it; do not make it wrong, and do not try to go to an 8.

Say to yourself: *I love you, I love you, I love you. It is okay to be at a two. Hello two. Here we are at two. I am willing to be here with you for these breaths.* Soften as you breathe. That lets the whole universe within you shift and lets you come to a higher space.

Where Is Your Energy Going?

Ask yourself when making choices or decisions, or just going about your day: *Am I doing this as means to an end, or am I doing this as the end itself?*

A client I worked with named Stephanie was deliberating about whether to leave her job. She did not like what she was doing and wanted to find something more purposeful, but she was afraid she would not make any money at that. Stephanie worried, if she honored herself, life would slam her down, and she would be stuck in a worse situation. When I felt into her system, I noted feelings of worthlessness and a fear of abandonment. We did the work together and allowed a major shift in her body that let fear go. We brought up these energies and she let unworthiness go. She let the tension where these energies had resided in her body release. She felt clear, relaxed, free, and at ease.

All of a sudden, she had total clarity about what do in her work situation. She got an idea for a completely different way to generate money, by doing jobs for friends and working as a personal assistant while building her business. It would more than recoup the money she was making in her job that was sucking all her time and energy and had her buying into lack consciousness. As soon as she shifted, a certainty and a knowing arose in her: *Life is on my side. I am always provided for. I am always taken care of.*

Stephanie had shifted her brain. Solutions came in; things made sense. Resources were evident. She felt great about the new choice and taking those steps to rearrange her life made it happen. She felt confident because she was in a heightened state of truly honoring herself in the equation. She had amazing new ideas for her business, which developed much more quickly than she imagined it would.

Stephanie was staying in her job so she would not have to feel that fear. She was living fear, but she did not have to *feel* it if she stayed in the *safe* job doing the *right* thing according to the mind and programming, even though it was destroying her health. The more she realized: *I am using this as a means to an end,* she thought: *If I stick at this job long enough, I will finally make enough money so I can take a year off and develop my business.* But even as those thoughts did bring temporary relief, she felt a fluttering tension in her stomach when she tuned into them.

Those thoughts were not true; Stephanie knew they were not her highest path. She instead honored what would feel light, what would feel free. Rearranging her job situation felt freeing. It was the end in and of itself. It was no longer a means to an end. She felt free being on her new path.

Whenever you make a choice—such as whether to take a medication, to see a particular practitioner, or to stay in a relationship or job—consider how you feel when you make that choice. Do you feel light? Do you feel supported? Do you feel inspired? All of these are evidence from your body feedback mechanism.

If you feel heaviness instead, that indicates it's not a true choice. If the mind says: *But I should just do it, and then I will be free,* or *If I do this, then something good will happen*—that's the conditionality. You feel it as a tension in your body, an anxiety or acceleration that feels uneasy. Trust those sensations because your body is your feedback device; it is showing you the path to the most abundance for you. Do not view those sensations as wrong, and do not overlook them. Soften and breathe into them and let them bring you the insight they have for you.

It may feel uneasy to see where you are buying into a lie such as: *You can't make money doing that* or *You do not deserve to have a better relationship,* so you keep trying to make the one you are in work. Pay attention to those sensations. They are going to show possibilities and solutions. It is all contained in the packet of the experience. Let the experience in, and you get the solutions included with it! You don't need to protect yourself from the experience. It's just energy moving through you. Breathe, enter into your body, open the packet, let it unfold, and it will show you all the solutions.

In the next chapter, I share the full process for instant healing. Now that you've practiced softening around the ideas and beliefs you used to hold more tightly, you've learned the value of surrender and have begun to let yourself go there, and you've begun to connect with the Source Intelligence that created you and courses through you, you are ready to activate infinite power within yourself.

CHAPTER SIX

Shift Your Consciousness to Shift Your Health – Your 3-Step Process for Instant Healing

As I have outlined in this book, you are made of pure energy. The factors at play are frequency and vibration. The practices you have been doing here allow your tendency to think of yourself as a physical, static, solid, separate entity to fall away. You are no longer operating in the paradigm of that idea or that reality. When you know your foundation is frequency and vibration, you come into a different way of being and can make instant and significant changes to create and manifest what you want.

Our ideas about scientific *truths* are constantly changing. People have seen the world as a finite thing with specific boundaries and firm edges; however, the science of quantum physics has shown what looks physical, solid, and unchanging is actually energy waves, interconnected and in constant flux. The more we have studied the smallest parts of our world, the more we understand that what we thought was true and absolute is more subjective than we thought. As we uncover greater and greater truths, it is wise to question and refine the new understandings as we embrace a new way. It is also wise to loosen up the old ones and let discovery and advancement bring us into a new dimension of our understanding.

TO CHANGE HEALTH, YOU MUST CHANGE CONSCIOUSNESS

Until you make a shift of consciousness, you are not changing anything. You may move the parts around; it may look different, but you do not experience more joy or more abundance or more freedom. Many people change their jobs or their relationships but then enter into a new job or a new relationship and, after a while, create the same situation again: *I left that marriage, and I left that job, and I left that person, but now I am with another person who is also narcissistic and abusive.* Or: *I made more money, but then I lost it all because XYZ happened.* People have moved across the country because they realize: *I have to change my health, and there is mold here; let me go where it is drier.* But they move to a new area and none of their health problems resolve, or one issue resolves but a new health problem comes up. There is no real change.

No matter how much you move around the parts to create a real shift in your experience of health, wealth, love, joy, or freedom, you must change your consciousness before anything higher can show up. When you first shift your consciousness, even just 2%, it always, always, *always* changes your reality. It changes your body. It changes your relationships. It changes your money. Unexpected, serendipitous things happen when you shift your consciousness.

After reading this far in the book, you are more ready to release any attachment to the outcome, so you can be fully present here, now. You are ready to shift your focus from the outer to the inner and let go of what seems to be happening on the outside. When you let go of attachment and outer focus, you are guaranteed to have power and abundance come in effortlessly.

Allow a new intention, a new aim of what you are going for. You're not going for the end result; you're aiming for the state of BE-ing that matches that end result.

Why do you want health, anyway?

So you feel good and feel grateful for life.

Why do you want more money?

So you feel free and can live freely.

Why do you want a great relationship?

So you feel loved and accepted unconditionally.

You've got to create that end result *first*. This is a new intention.

Instead of a Have-Do-Be mindset, in which we think: *If only I could* **have** *my health*—or money, or a relationship—*then I could* **do** *the things I need to do, and then I would* **be** *happy*, you have to reverse that.

As I shared in *The MindBody Toolkit*, we must remember Be-Do-Have: *When I am in that fulfilled state of* **be***ing, I automatically* **do** *the things that match that state, and then I* **have** *my health*—or money, or relationship.

Are you willing to get into that state of BE-ing even before anything has changed?

Release the circumstances and conditions you think are required because until you move into the consciousness of freedom and well-being, it cannot be created in your physical body. When you focus on the *Having*, trying to have a particular thing so you can then be happy, you miss the point. That would be off in the future, not here, now. You can't create it that way. You must enter the state of BE-ing first, regardless of what you have or don't have; that's the only way ignition happens.

If you wait until you find a better job or make more money, so that you will feel freer to take inspired action or follow your heart, it can never happen, because you are still in the consciousness of fear and poverty or lack. You may create more money. You may create a different situation, but it will not create more freedom. It will not create more joy until you shift your consciousness. Let go of the outer attachment and focus instead on the inner shift of feeling more peace now, feeling more freedom now, even feeling 2% more at ease now, and let go of any outer things you think need to happen. This will allow all of the outer things to come into your perfect alignment and manifestation.

Health and Wealth: They Are Connected

Your health is determined by your frequency. When you are in a state of joy, love, or gratitude, it affects your cells. It affects your neurochemicals. It affects your DNA. Your cells are affected by your consciousness and your frequency. Make it your priority to address your state of being and choose a state of peace. Choose a state of ease. Soften your shoulders and release stress, no matter what is happening. Situations will resolve themselves. Resources will appear out of nowhere. You will get a phone call from someone you've been wanting to connect with but didn't know how to reach.

Let Life serve you in unexpected ways because you have prioritized your inner state of well-being. This allows real health, wealth, and abundance to arrive instead of pseudo-health, in which one disease resolves, but another one crops up. Maybe your life gets easier, and you have more energy, but then something falls apart and there are ten more things you have to take care of. It is like the whack-a-mole game where you have to whack a little mole back into its hole over and over, and another crops up as soon as you get one in place. You think you are getting somewhere, but you are really just staying busy in the same frequency and consciousness. You have only moved around the parts.

Maybe you attain pseudo-wealth and make lots of money, but you're working your butt off and sacrificing your health to do it. Or maybe you make a lot of money, but an unexpected expense appears, so you have not created wealth or freedom. Or maybe you find a new job, and you make more money, but you are busy all the time and miserable because you are overwhelmed, and you do not have the relationships you want or the peace of mind you want.

Did you create true wealth?

True health, true wealth, and true abundance are always, always a shift in frequency; they are not physical, external situations or circumstances. When you remember you have the key to powerful manifestation, you let go of the old path. You see abundance, health, and peace are all connected to what is in you.

We tend to compartmentalize our life: Over here is my health. Over there is my money. Over there is my relationship, social life, or home. Even if there is improvement in one area, your consciousness dictates the overall picture. You may have more flow with your money, but then you have no time to enjoy it because you are working all the time. You may have a job you love but your relationships suffer, and you don't have real connections because you're working all the time, or you're grouchy at the end of the workday. The compartments may look like something good is happening, but that is offset by an emptiness somewhere else, and that is evidence you have not shifted your frequency.

Many people spend their whole life moving the parts around. This is going well but that is going poorly. Then finally this other thing that was going so poorly is going well. You are constantly dealing with the same levels of frustration, lack, or overwhelm. That is not an actual shift into true health, wealth, or abundance. Shifting your consciousness first *does* create a real expansion, and it will be an expansion in every sector of your life.

Real Fulfillment Versus Chasing Fear and the False-Self

The small-self, or false-self, is going to tell you that you can't possibly be at peace until you have your health back, you need to have money before you can be free and do what you love, or you're no prize package—you can't leave this relationship and have real love. The false-self is always going to keep you busy. It's going to make things conditional.

Do a little check-in with yourself:

- What are your three highest priorities?

- Do they bring you a sense of joy thinking about them, holding them in your intention?

- Are they a means to an end or are they True-Self desires?

From this awareness, write five intentions you truly would like to manifest.

- Look at each and list *why* you want it.

- Is this item the actual end itself, or is it a means to get what you truly desire?

If any one of them is a means to an end, it is the false-self telling you that once you get that thing then you will be happy, then you will be free, then you will have more peace. It's an illusion to keep you busy not noticing that you aren't getting anywhere.

I invite you to erase the chalkboard of all those conditions, all those things you think you need before you feel free or happy and which leave you begging to connect with the essence of freedom or the essence of joy or the essence of peace.

If you have picked one of these now and welcomed it, familiarize yourself with what that feels like. It makes it infinitely easier to welcome this experience into your life if you practice into the experience first.

Take a few minutes a day and connect with what it would feel like if you did have that perfect job, or all the money you could ever want. What would it feel like if you did have your greatest lover and best friend who loves you unconditionally?

Let the essence of this in because this is what creates a consciousness shift. This is what creates a cellular shift. This is what creates an electromagnetic shift, and this is exactly what invites and allows everything you are asking for to come into your life.

Always go into the real fulfillment as compared with chasing away fear, trying to escape, or trying to get something so that you will then be fulfilled.

You're Just Trying to Get High

The truth is that everything you are looking for is only a way for you to get higher vibrationally, for you to feel freer, for you to feel more joy, for you to feel more love. But it can't happen from the outside in; it can only happen from the inside out.

Your body is the technology that creates it. The language of the creative field is *feeling*. When you feel the frequency in your body, you have generated an electromagnetic shift and begun to generate the chemical shifts—*physical* events within you. You've got to feel the frequency of what you're asking for in order for it to arise in your physical life. You don't need to wait for it to show up in the physical realm before you generate the experience within you. You generate it, then it shows up. Here's how to get to the energy underneath those desires:

- Make a list of everything you could ever ask for.

- Review the list, and ask yourself *why* you want those things; for example:

  Why do I want to have more friends or an awesome social circle of like-minded people who understand me?

  Why do I want to have meaningful, purposeful work I love where I can express myself?

  Why do I want to have robust, vibrant health and high energy?

You want those things so you can feel a certain way, so you can live a certain way, so you can be what you are truly here to be, your True Self. But what if you do not need any condition to start expressing the True Self right here, right now, as you are? It takes forgiveness for not feeling as high as you would like to feel right now, forgiveness for circumstances not being the way you would ideally like them to be, forgiveness for being in a relationship that does not honor you.

Be willing to feel a sense of peace with yourself right now anyway.

> *We are not here only to manifest our heart's every desire and get what we want. We are here, especially within the third density plane of existence, to learn how to make the choice to love unconditionally within the very convincing illusion of separation.*
> ~ Ziad Masri, *Reality Unveiled*

Even if you have discomfort in your body or excruciating physical pain, soften anyway and let in the experience.

What if, despite the physical or even emotional pain, you are willing to be 2% more at peace with yourself right now?

You can only create more of what you already have. If you decide there is even a 2% increase, a tiny little spark of peace you are willing to feel despite your pain or circumstances, and you choose to feel love, the light will come into your now moment. It will come into your body right now, come into your consciousness right now. This allows everything physical, mental, and emotional to shift.

Remember everything you could ever want, everything you could ever ask for is so you can feel the essence and the lightness and the vibrancy of who you are. Then reverse-engineer these ideals and let yourself feel them right here, right now, where you are, as you are, how you are. This is how you activate conscious creation.

Make a list now of all the ways you get to feel and all the things you get to experience when those conditions are met.

Can you feel the frequency of it? Can you embody these feelings and experiences in your body right here now?

Now make a list of everything you think is *in the way* of you embodying this state *as if it were here right now*.

Examples:

- *I can't feel gratitude because I have so much pain.*

- *I can't feel and be free because there is too much to do, and I'm overwhelmed.*

- *I can't feel well because I'm exhausted and have to keep going.*

- *I can't feel this because I don't know how.*

Are you willing to see these statements are not actually *true*?

You can keep letting them be true, but they're the program talking, not you.

Will you keep identifying as the program or are you ready to reclaim your power?

What comes up for you when I say these words?

If you are willing to see these statements are not actually true, you are ready to go on to the next step.

The Swamp Exercise

If you are not, I invite you to do the *Swamp Exercise*. It's a powerful exercise I use in my Embracing Health group, so we get the mucky energy out and let it dissolve.

Set aside ten to thirty minutes and write down every thought and feeling you have right now about why you can't heal, why you can't be powerful, and why your heart's desires cannot be met.

Start with "I swamp" and write all the thoughts and ideas the small-self has to say that feel true. Know it's the small-self purging and give them space to just have at it. Fill up as much as you can of the whole page with what this part of you has to say. Go as deep, dark, and mucky as you possibly can.

Examples:

I swamp . . .

- I'll never make it.

- I can't do this.

- Nothing I do will matter.

- It's hopeless.

- I try and try, and nothing will ever work.

- This stuff is crap.

Write everything you fear, everything in there. Nothing is too dark to bring into the light.

When you are done, hold the page to your heart and say, "Thank you for letting me see all these thoughts and feelings that were held inside me. I am willing to love you and set you free."

INCREASING YOUR FREQUENCY AND THE SCALE OF CONSCIOUSNESS

In physical terms, energy takes the form of frequency and vibration. Different frequencies have different qualities. Lower frequencies are heavier and dense. We feel emotions of powerlessness, fear, anger, or frustration. Thoughts at these frequencies may be: *I'll never make it*, or *I have to keep going*.

Higher frequencies are lighter. We may feel the emotions of love, joy, or gratitude, which is a very high frequency. The body will feel more fluid, uplifted, and energized at a higher frequency.

This has been mapped in a quantitative way in the work of David Hawkins, MD, who demonstrated how emotions correlate with vibrational frequencies.

Go to DrKimD.com/BYOHbonuses to view the Map of Consciousness.

It does not mean that guilt, grief, or fear are negative or bad; they are simply lower frequencies. They may be harder to embrace and move through, so we resist and or suppress them. This is where the damage comes. The energy that goes into suppression costs us. All the energy that could be going into manifesting our heart's desire gets consumed because it takes a lot of energy to keep from feeling those dense emotions. The energies and frequencies of acceptance, love, joy, and peace feel lighter, and it is easier to embrace them and move through them.

I want to point out right up front that it's all energy. It's not good or bad. It is not about toxic energy or therapeutic energy. It is about the energy we tend to resist and the energy we move through more easily and tend to embrace. If we could welcome all energy, then everything would move through us. Our emotions would move through within seconds, and it would be a fluid experience of different aspects of life. We would maintain a vibrant state of health.

We instead tend to resist these lower frequency energies because of the mind. They are uncomfortable, and we think they'll last forever, or we make them wrong and shameful. Or they are inconvenient, so we save them for later and stuff the emotions in the body, and disease gets created. We haven't learned to be in flow with emotions and energy, so we resist life. We resist ourselves.

The Scale of Consciousness

David Hawkins, MD, was a physician who understood everything is energy. He dedicated his life's work to mapping out these states of consciousness. He did a vast amount of research on the energy body and the frequency of emotions. His work mathematically quantified energy states in the body, and what those vibrations do to the body, such as what happens when you suppress grief and hold that energy in your system.

Grief is a lower-frequency emotion. When we suppress it, it's toxic to the body. It doesn't have to be. It can be profoundly opening. Grief can deepen our capacity for compassion, connection, love, and joy. But grief, like other emotions, is meant to move through and move out. It's not meant to stick around for years or decades while we put an inordinate amount of energy into suppressing it.

How does it end up doing this?

We may have disconnected from our hearts and don't know how to move through grief. Maybe someone died, and you have never fully mourned. You're sure it will kill you if you were to really let it all in. It's just too big. You keep yourself busy; you do not talk about it. You don't go to the grave site. Maybe it's hard during the holidays, but the rest of the year you kind of plug on and get through. You have grief in your system *all the time* though it isn't felt, but it certainly hasn't gone anywhere. It's mostly unconscious, but it is still affecting your body all the time. It gets triggered in certain situations. It may be dormant, but it's always there. It's always affecting you, even when you aren't triggered, and you don't feel it.

The research by Dr. Hawkins' team shared, in his book *Power vs. Force,* looked specifically at how this suppressed energy affects cells, DNA, the brain, and overall functioning. They were able to see how deeply our health is related to the energies and emotions we hold. They mapped how our state of health is related to our vibrational frequency. We can quantify someone's overall frequency and give them a reading of where, as a human energy system, they are calibrating.

None of this is to judge you. It's not a way to try to get to a higher level. It's information to help you understand how your energy system works. The lower states of shame, guilt, apathy, grief, and fear are dense states to embody. Suppressing those kinds of emotions is toxic to your body. It will keep you at a low frequency and prevent your brain from seeing possibilities or creating inspired solutions. No matter how positive you try to be, until you actually release these energies, they will cause limitation in your life. Situations will continually come up in which you find you're not free; there are no solutions; it's not a win-win situation; you always lose—situations will repeatedly try to bring up those old emotions.

You can get a sense of where in yourself this may be happening if you examine what's happening in your life right now. Look at the biggest challenge you are facing. How does it make you feel? If you're harboring dense emotions, you feel angry or bummed out about what's happening. You're busy and overwhelmed and do not see a way out. You'll have things coming up that are scary and threatening. You'll feel like a victim of your circumstances.

Being in higher frequency also affects your outlook. You will see that life is happening *for* you. You will experience challenges as opportunities for growth. You will embrace life and move forward more fluidly when you have released lower, dense energies.

The calibration studies Dr. Hawkins performed show that your vibrational frequency directly impacts how you feel emotionally, your level of health physically, your mood, how you see the world, and even your external circumstances and external reality. The research shows that most of this was not conscious, meaning energies were below the level of the conscious mind. Your body is responding to everything around you and registering a certain frequency.

Some people think disease processes are unavoidable with aging. They are not; disease develops when you harbor low-density emotions and do not clear them up. Over the years, they become more deleterious to your health and cause more disease. Disease is caused not by the aging process, but by how long you have been carrying toxic energies and emotions.

Your energy field registers information your conscious mind is not aware of. In muscle testing, the system goes weak if something is harmful, and strong if it is healthful. For example, if a person were holding a vial containing a toxin, their energy would register this signal and go weak, even though they had no idea consciously what was in the vial. Their energy system registers that low frequency, demonstrating, on some level, the electromagnetic system senses what it is encountering.

We are continuously registering electromagnetic information. Our system lets us know anything we're seeking information about. Some people may have a gut feeling that signals them to make a specific choice. As they tune in, they find that sensation is guiding them to better and better situations, sometimes about information they could not possibly have known from the conscious mind alone. We can tune into this guidance for pretty much everything—from what foods will nurture us most to whether we should move forward with a relationship.

However, most people have learned not to pay attention to this kind of information. They have been taught overtly or covertly to rely only on the rational mind and the information they've arrived at through rational thinking. How much we miss when we try to live that way. How much awareness we block that we could be accessing to live our lives in flow.

Our system knows which people are life-giving for us and which are not beneficial for us to be around. Our bodies are affected by the bodies around us. We can receive uplifting and harmonious energy by being around certain people. It strengthens our body and health.

The opposite is also true. In lower frequencies, like states of shame, guilt, and grief, we suck up and consume more energy than we are creating and contributing. That is why when you are around certain people, they feel like energy vampires. Their system depletes your energy if you keep choosing to participate. It is exhausting to be around them because they suck up energy from others around them. People who complain or tell their sob story or always need somebody else to listen to their plight are doing that. They will wear one person out and move on to the next friend and start telling them their story.

At first, you might feel bad or pity them, give them more attention, or try to help them, but you eventually realize your contribution is not helping them. They never do anything functional with it; they never get on their own feet. They keep using the energy of everyone around them yet stay in their low state. In relationships like that, it's best to walk the other way. Love them, wish them well, and move into your own space because that relationship is not going to benefit you, and they are not using the energy in a way that will be a contribution to them. This is what love would do.

On the opposite end of the spectrum, there are people in higher states of consciousness who bring you into a higher alignment. Being around them lifts you up, makes you feel more alive, and makes you feel more positive and joyful. They are contributing energy to the world because they are tapped into the wholeness, the infinite source within. The effect of these individuals alters your brainwave patterning in beneficial ways. You may suddenly have insights you did not have before. Solutions appear where there had been none. When people around us are in those higher frequencies and higher states, it is contagious.

Our orthodontist is this kind of person. After being in the waiting room for my first appointment, I had about ten brilliant ideas for my business. I felt uplifted, joyful, and empowered, and I enjoyed my time there. It wasn't until after the second time this happened I realized it was about the harmonics of the space and the energy of this amazing man who holds so much love in his heart. It happens every time I've been to his office, and I've also seen this same effect in my kids' systems. It's unusually powerful. Interestingly, I found out more recently he had gone through a profound hardship with the death of his adult child. He shared this with vulnerability and love in his heart. This is the radical healing effect that happens when we keep our heart open and let our deepest grief open us to even deeper love. We become a healing presence in the world.

Your Consciousness Equals Your Reality

The scale of consciousness, which coincides with the emotional state we are in, is calibrated in a logarithmic way, meaning we go exponentially higher physically as we come into an even slightly higher state emotionally. This scale has been numbered so we can quantify the states in relation to each other. The lowest level on the scale of human consciousness is ten to the 20th power: shame. The numbers are logarithmic, not linear, so level 20 indicates 10 to the 20th power. The highest level on the scale of human consciousness is 1,000—$10^{1,000}$ or 10 to the 1,000th power—which matches *Christ Consciousness*, also called *Oneness Consciousness*. At that level, we are no longer

Be Your Own Healer

identified with the small-self and are entirely embodying the consciousness of the True Self.

An image of Dr. Hawkins' Map of Consciousness can be found in the bonus section that accompanies this book at DrKimD.com/BYOHbonuses.

In the lower levels, as I mentioned, we consume more energy than we contribute. When we're suppressing so many densities, it takes more energy to run our system than what we are generating within ourselves. However, as consciousness rises to the level of 200—10 to the 200th power—we begin to contribute more energy than we are consuming. There are two big inflection points on this scale as we come from the lower, denser frequencies into the higher, lighter frequencies. These occur at 200 and 500 on the scale of consciousness.

At the frequency of 200—10 to the 200th power—we move beyond fear and step into *Courage*. From the state of courage, we are more connected with the heart, the strength that comes from the *heart chakra*, the energy center around the heart. Courage is when we choose to open even when life throws us challenges. For example, even if you are sick or have been given a cancer prognosis, you are willing to open and to receive what life has for you. Even though a situation may be hard, you are willing to hold the space that something higher may be possible.

Courage is also present when we're willing to go beyond our fear. For example, it takes an immense amount of courage to question our current paradigm, the current *reality* of other people's speech and actions, and to open to a new possibility that we do not already understand.

You are finding courage to read this book and continue when it may be shaking things up for you, or it may be confusing at times to integrate something different. This courage is a powerful inflection point where you transcend fear and come into something lighter. Fear no longer controls you and limits your decisions. This can't happen when you reside below the level of courage.

Questioning things takes courage and is important. For true healing to happen, we must open beyond what we already understand and can control. Venturing into the unknown seems risky to the mind. People can be controlled by fear when they have not yet found courage. Teaching people not to question authority is one way a populace can be kept under control. Doctors are taught not to question the status quo. Skepticism of new ideas is seen as a strength in the conventional medical culture. To say, "I don't know" is a weakness. Doctors are supposed to have the answers and understand the body fully. No wonder there have been so many people staying sick and finding no real solutions in that system.

What we *do* understand about the body is infinitesimally small compared to what we *do not* understand. It's okay to acknowledge that, but in the current paradigm it takes courage. Behind that doorway, in the not-knowing, lie new possibilities. We open to let in new ideas, new perspectives, new possibilities. We enter the unknown and are beyond the conclusions. We become curious and open-minded. This is when the best ideas and solutions come in.

Above level 200, the body has the energy to heal itself. It has extra energy beyond what you use to function moment to moment. Solutions come in. You may finally have the courage to leave an abusive relationship. As soon as you take that step, the resources appear. Maybe you take a step into the unknown, and then have an idea about how you could sustain yourself financially that had not occurred to you before. That courage lets your body work differently, lets your brain work differently, lets your body have more energy, and lets creative solutions come into your life.

Don't wait until fear isn't there before you find courage and choose yourself. You are the only one who can choose to live from courage when you are feeling fear.

At level 500—10 to the 500th power—is *Love*. This one is powerful because we enter a new level of functionality and possibility. Dr. Hawkins' research shows that even the greatest thinkers and people who famously contributed to the world were still functioning below 500. They were functioning from a place of *Reason*—10 to the 400th power. These great thinkers, including Albert Einstein, were found to calibrate in the high 400s, but always below the level of Love. Reason is a higher sense of what is *right*, which comes from the mind and is based in judgment and fairness. We may do good for others because we understand it is ultimately going to come back to us; however, we are still functioning from this mind and from judgment.

Love, sitting at 500 on the Hawkins scale, is higher than Reason. Love is something we cannot understand from the mind. Love is choosing to give even though it does not seem to make sense. Love is choosing to follow the lightness in your heart even when you do not understand why.

Love is choosing to change your situation, leave a relationship, or start a new business venture, even when everyone else says it won't work. You feel the lightness, you feel the acceleration, you feel a deep inner knowing, and you follow it. You say yes, and then you gain exponentially more power. That is why it is so powerful. At the level of Love or above, the body will reverse disease. The body can no longer harbor disease and will begin healing itself in the frequency of 540—10 to the 540th power—or above. This is also why, when you soften your shoulders and breathe into your heart to let higher consciousness in, something happens that comes from a higher space. You do not already understand it. It goes beyond reason, but you do it anyway. New awareness will come in, and yes, it will ultimately make sense, but you have to first open your heart before that can happen.

Choose Love, even before you understand why, then the understanding can come, and things later make sense. You've entered a higher mind-state that can understand this. In the lower states, these things do not make any sense. We must choose first.

This is why, at the beginning of all my group calls and sessions, we drop in to release the high-beta brainwave functioning and come into a slow-beta or alpha brainwave frequency. A person will block out everything I'm saying when they remain in their beta programming.

When we first open their system, love can go in and new information can go in. They let in the higher Truth because they are receptive. Always, when you want to share truth with someone, *relax your body first.* Come into a higher state, and you are already communicating the transmission of consciousness you're intending to share. This allows *their* system to relax and open, and then there could be a conversation that is fruitful.

At the level of Love and above, you start creating at all-new levels, doing things other people cannot imagine, and they will not know how you do it. You will have synchronicities come in that are inexplicable and serve a great purpose in your life. You will be in flow and feel the lightness physically, mentally, and emotionally. You will witness miracles happening in your material reality. In the frequency of Love or above, things happen to you that do not seem to happen for other people because you are no longer subjected to the rules they're living under. Blessings come in, and you are taken care of. When you are willing to reside in the frequency of Love or above, you are living in majesty.

Small Consciousness Shifts Equal Exponential Quantum Shifts

When there is even a small shift in consciousness, it translates to an exponentially large shift in your life. You can take comfort in knowing that although it may take some energy to shift your consciousness, you *can* move a mountain. Maybe you have been feeling depressed for many, many years, and neurological patterns keep it in place. Maybe you have harbored a victim viewpoint that life is happening *to* you, and it is so unfair, so you are fighting and fighting and staying in fight-or-flight mode.

You have seen what happens when you live only from fear and closure. You haven't yet begun to see what happens when you live from Love.

Maybe there are old patterns with money or relationships that have always been bad and have never been okay. It can shift. It may be a little uncomfortable in the beginning because you are not used to the new frequency. You're creating a shift in millions of neural networks that have been put in place. It may feel a little slow in the beginning because you are not seeing the results, but it is a well-invested venture to learn to shift your frequency because even the slightest shift in your frequency creates a massive exponential shift in your physical reality.

One of the things in Dr. Hawkins' research I find so fascinating as a doctor is that, when we get up into the higher frequencies of Love or above, we begin to heal cellular disease. The red blood cells that have had jagged edges from cellular and genetic damage start to smooth out; they are not so sticky. There is less inflammation, things are flowing better, and health is strengthened. As we go higher, this effect is faster and more significant. In fact, for a person at an energy field calibrating at the level of *Peace* and above, which is 600, disease cannot exist.

This means, if only for a moment, you harbor a sense of Peace, unconditional self-acceptance, fully cultivated presence, the state of *I am willing to be exactly where I am as I am and how I am*; it has a potent and *immediate* effect on cellular healing. This is why individuals like Mother Teresa, who calibrated at a level above 600, could walk through the impoverished streets of Calcutta, where most people would run the other way because it is so depressing and so horrifying, and share blessings that helped people heal. She maintained a very high frequency of light and love and health even in a very low-frequency environment and brought that light and healing to other people.

I have approached my practice in medicine by focusing on *shifting the consciousness*, first mine, then others', in order to shift the physical. It's not a linear growth curve; it's an exponential growth curve. I know the leverage we have when we do this and how even subtle shifts in consciousness have massive and vast impacts on every aspect of our health.

A 3-STEP PROCESS FOR INSTANT HEALING

I hope by now you have become more adept at focusing attention on your personal frequency and have gotten on board for setting your primary intention on shifting your frequency. No matter what is happening in your life, and no matter what you want to create, let go and surrender, so you enter a higher state. This is the way to allow an instant shift, and this is the way to allow a new manifestation. I've cultivated many ways to do this, but the most essential step is that you gain your power back. What you are asking for cannot happen until you have cultivated more power.

When I was sick, I had already learned a ton of information about MindBody Medicine and how the body heals itself, but I kept wondering how to do it: *This is great to understand, but how do I activate healing? What do I do?* It wasn't going to come from learning more. I had to cultivate the power within myself. I had to *let in the experience* rather than resist it. I had to let the experience show me.

Your system has the capacity to learn from experience.

It's not enough to understand how this works; you must allow an embodiment. You've got to open your energy centers—soften your body, relax, and breathe—for that to happen. All the head knowledge in the world will not do it. You've got to bring it into the body. That can't happen when you are tight, when you are closed, when you—the small-self you—are in control.

There are many ways to do this, but the foundation of all of them is what I call the Instant Elevation Technique. This technique is instant because you are creating an immediate quantum shift which instantly registers in your electromagnetic field. Over time, this translates to physical, chemical shifts and the shifting of outer circumstances, but at the level of the electromagnetics it is instant. You are elevating because you are increasing your frequency and increasing your consciousness. Your cells are always listening. They are at your service, standing by like little soldiers ready to operate, create, and transmit at the frequency you choose, at the frequency you reside in.

After healing myself, people would ask me, "How do you do it?" I had to check in with my own system to really listen and break down this process so I could teach others. *What am I doing? Where is my attention going? What am I doing with my body?* There was a specific 3-step process that was always happening which allowed me to cultivate the power and put it into manifestation to create change. It was an instant shift into a higher frequency so I called it the Instant Elevation.

Remember, the only two things you have any control over are *where you put your attention* and *what you do with your body*. Everything else is a delusion. You think you have control over your kids. You think you have control over your diet. You think you have control over your money. Forget it. You do not have control over anything other than where you put your attention and what you do with your body. Leverage where you *are* in charge, where you *do* have power and potency and use that for the purpose of increasing your frequency and consciousness.

The ABCs of the 3-Step Process

The three steps to the Instant Elevation Technique are:

- Awareness

- Breathing

- Choice

Having been trained as an emergency medicine doctor working in trauma, I was under a lot of pressure, and algorithms—which are basically a go-to memorized sequence—are helpful in those circumstances. ABC in that case meant Airway, Breathing, Circulation, so I didn't have to think and be creative. In an emergency, I could go right to that cue. Following the ABCs, doctors first check to see if a person has an intact airway to get oxygen through. Then we check whether they are actively breathing. Third, we assess their circulation. Do they have a pulse? Is blood circulating through their body?

If those steps are done out of order, life is at stake. Imagine you see someone gushing blood from a wound and become distracted. You immediately focus on addressing the bleeding only later to realize the person had a blocked airway or wasn't breathing. Whatever you do for step C will be in vain until you first address A and B. The same is true with the Instant Elevation.

So many people let their attention get pulled to the gushing blood. They're scrambling to address that, putting all of their energy into that, then wondering why there's no oxygen, no lifeforce coming through. They never brought in awareness of what was truly needed in the situation. Their energy gets wasted because they're missing the big picture. When you are triggered or struggling, go to the ABCs.

A go-to algorithm helped me with my energy consciousness. When I would become aware of stress, fear, tension, or an overall heaviness that indicated my frequency was low, I needed a go-to process. When I am in that low frequency, I cannot remember the higher concepts, I cannot hear Divine guidance. I feel so disconnected, confused, and scared. But if I use this ABC tool, I can immediately find my way back. And like in the Emergency Room, the sequence is important.

A: Awareness

Cultivate your awareness. This is the most important step, the most powerful one, and if you forget the other two steps, the main shift happens here. You've been practicing this throughout this book. When you bring your awareness into the here and now, you have power. Your body only lives in the now. It cannot live in the past. It cannot live in the future. It cannot live in the outer projection of what you think reality is. It can only live in the now. Bring your attention into the physical body.

Place your hand on your heart. Bring your shoulders up and then drop them down and feel and sense your body. It will access you to the now.

I have shared an audio file called "The Instant Elevation Technique" in the free book bonuses.

Go to DrKimD.com/BYOHbonuses and relax as I guide you in integrating this process for yourself.

You will practice bringing your awareness back into the body, back into the here and now.

Whenever you notice you are in a low-frequency state or notice you are dealing with circumstances that do not seem to be budging, no matter what you do, remember ABC. Let increasing your frequency be your focus. Bring your awareness back to your body. If you close your eyes and breathe, you can sense your energy coming back into your body from wherever it may be, releasing and erasing the chalkboard of everything and everyone around you.

B: Breathing

Shift your breathing. When you are in lower frequency states and survival mode, the sympathetic nervous system turns on and your breath becomes shallow and fast. The breath is coming into the upper lung fields, and you are using accessory muscles of inspiration, which are your neck and shoulder muscles, and that creates tension. Your brain focuses into small-minded thinking, so you can't access big-picture awareness. Your body shunts blood to the working muscles and away from digestion, immune function, and other housekeeping activities that restore health. This sympathetic nervous system activation, or fight-or-flight state, is helpful for short-term emergencies, but is not a functional way to live your life. You are wasting energy, and you are not moving oxygen and nutrients throughout your body.

Bring your shoulders up to your ears and take a deep breath. Then exhale as you let your shoulders relax. You will begin breathing more into your belly. Relax your shoulders and see the breath coming all the way down to the lower lung field. Let the belly balloon out with the inhales, and let it sink back with exhales.

When you switch your breathing, it switches your nervous system. It turns off the sympathetic nervous system, the fight-or-flight system, and it turns on the parasympathetic nervous system, which is the relax-and-restore system. By shifting your breathing, you ignite that. Let the belly balloon out with the inhale; let the belly settle back in with the exhale. If this does not come easily at first, it may be because you have been living in fight-or-flight mode for a long time. With a little practice, the body will eventually adjust to what you are asking it to do.

Give the body the image to show it what you are asking. Picture a big red balloon in the belly and pelvis, expanding out with the inhale and settling back with the exhales. Your mind works in terms of images, and it gets the picture and lets go of tension it is holding and activates breathing in a new way.

After bringing awareness to your body, breathing is your second step. Anytime you notice you are contracted, in a low frequency, or feeling contraction about circumstances in your life that are not working out, no matter what you do, switch your breathing to activate the parasympathetic nervous system and let it go to work for you.

C: Choice

Choose consciously. When you are in the sympathetic nervous system fight-or-flight space—those lower frequencies of fear, grief, or guilt—you are not in conscious choice. Your unconscious automated programs take over. You are going to be destructive. You may eat things that are not good for your body, snap at someone you love, mess up at work, and wonder why your life is such a mess. Your choices are coming from your unconscious.

You must shift your frequency to make choices that align with your True-Self. Once you bring attention and energy to the present moment, and bring your awareness into your body, you are in the now. You've come into the place of power. You have shifted your breathing out of the fight or flight nervous system, the sympathetic response that can only create more chaos and inflammation. You have shifted into the parasympathetic nervous system, which is the relaxation response that restores your body. You are no longer functioning from the unconscious. You have access to conscious choice.

If the only thing you do is intend: *I choose to live fully. I choose to love and accept myself. I choose to allow my frequency to rise. I choose to release fear and grief,* that is enough. The first two steps are essential because until you cultivate power, nothing you intend is going to be activated. That is why people can do affirmations over and over, but they are not in a frequency where those can take hold and be activated. This is why so many people do so much self-healing and personal development work and don't see major change. They've made a choice, but they haven't first shifted their consciousness. They haven't cultivated their power. The first two parts of this equation are the most important. When you have cultivated that power, it is unlimited, and what you can manifest in your life becomes infinite.

Let this step be very simple. Intention is enough. Surrender the small-self so you choose, act, and live from the True-Self. That intention is enough of a conscious choice.

> *God is awareness. So when we tune into our awareness,*
> *we close the space between the individual and God.*
> ~ Ram Das

Integration Exercise 4: Activate Instant Healing With the Instant Elevation Technique

You are now ready to begin practicing Instant Elevation as it was truly intended.

Awareness. Bring all of your attention, energy, and power *here*, now, into your body. Call it home from wherever it was, known and unknown.

You may see it off in the future, trying to make sure things go a certain way, or make sure things don't go wrong. Just erase the chalkboard of the future, blow away the chalk dust, and see all of the energy that is *your* energy come home now into your body. The only place you have any power to create the future is here, now in your body.

Next you may see some of it in the past, ruminating over what did or did not happen, holding resentment or anger, holding regret. Just let that go; erase the chalkboard of the past and welcome all your energy back home, now, into your body. The only place where you can resolve the past and come back to power is here, now, in your body.

You may notice some of your energy feels off with other people, monitoring what they need, tuning into how they feel, registering who they need you to be—helping them, saving them, or vesting yourself in being what you think they need. Just let that all go, erase the chalkboard of other people, blow away the chalk dust. Welcome your energy home in your body now. The only place you can truly connect with and contribute to others is right here, now, within your body.

Next, welcome any energy that may have gotten caught up in the ideas about yourself—who you are supposed to be, your traits and characteristics, your identity. This is the personal-self who has certain roles, achievements, a degree or the lack of a degree you think you need, all the ideas you have about who you think you are, and just let them go. Erase the chalkboard of this identity, blow away the chalk dust, and welcome the energy that is you, back home, here, now, in your body. The only place you will access your true power and capabilities, which are infinitely beyond any of those identities, is here, now, in your body.

Be willing to welcome all of your power, your presence right here, right now, letting your body be a portal through which to ground it.

Breath. Bring your breath through your heart, all the way down through your belly and pelvis. See it expanding out. Relax your shoulders and let go. Allow the breath to expand the belly out with the inhales. Let the belly sink back in with the exhales. Feel the flow of the breath. It's free, it's abundant. You will always have all the breath you ever need, now and in every now that comes. The breath is only in the now. Let in the moment with your sensation of the smooth, fluid breath. See the breath coming all the way down to your pelvis and expanding out like a big red balloon. Bring your awareness down the body and out through this area. Let the breath flow through all the hurts, all the pains, all the resentments, all the fears. Let it flow through any densities you have been holding, known and unknown.

Now allow *light* to come in with each breath and let it clear your system back to love and peace. See it as crystalline, Divine, pure, white light and let it just come through with the breath. See this white light expand through all the densities you've held, known and unknown, and clarify them all back to pure love.

Next bring *love* in with the light and with the breath. Welcome everything here with that love and peace and let your body receive this love with the breath. Let this love, this light, this breath move through all areas known and unknown where you have not known peace, where you have not known love, where you have held densities because you have not known truth.

See the breath expanding beyond you to let this love and peace emanate out beyond your being. Let it include everything that you are, known and unknown.

Choice. Cultivate conscious choice. Choose to live from Source Consciousness. Intend to connect with the space beyond All That Is, the space of Creator that is beyond the created. Let this space be what you are tuning into. *It* is what you allow yourself to be. Let this space be who you are; it is you, and you choose to let this space course through you. Let this space show you everything you need. Surrender your small-self choice to this Creator space so that you receive Healing, Intelligence, and Light. You can say out loud or to yourself: *I choose to know Truth and True Wholeness. I choose to live as the True Power and Light that I AM.*

I have an audio version of this process for you in the book bonuses.

Go to DrKimD.com/BYOHbonuses to listen as I guide you through this process.

Practice this regularly, and you will integrate the ability to activate this process within moments. Begin using this full version of the Instant Elevation Technique as your Daily Integration Exercise from here forward.

Make this practice your own. Surrender to it. Trust it. It is up to you whether you cultivate true power and allow the creation of your majestic life, or you give that power to the doubt and the fear and stay in the small-self longer. Eventually, you will make the choice to return to Who You Are.

When you do, it will require the release of the small-self, thinking mind who can never truly manifest anything. It will require a surrender to the Truth within you. Below is a quote that was very powerful for me during this process of surrendering in my medical practice. It's from the founder of osteopathic medicine, who had to follow his inner truth, letting go of everything the medical establishment said was true, and choose to let in a higher truth and a higher creation, which he very certainly did.

> *Know you are right and do your work accordingly.*
> ~ A.T. Still, MD, DO

I posted the above quote on the wall of my osteopathic medical office, where I treated hundreds of patients and witnessed amazing healings. Every time I read it, it reminded me to let go of what I think and let the healing come through me. I know we can do this, and my intention is that you choose to know as well.

Once you integrate this, your mind-body system will already know what you are asking it to do. Then you can do it in seconds, anytime, anywhere. Give yourself plenty of time and go slow with learning this. It's a subtle process, and you will see your body begin to show you how to make this your own.

Once you learn to master your energy, clear your field, and cultivate your power for healing and manifestation, you realize that the outer world, your lifestyle, occupation, and relationships may not be entirely supportive to your clarified heightened state. It's okay. Awareness is enough to let things begin to rearrange so your outer life and lifestyle support and sustain you living as the True-Self.

You can let things fall away, change them, or embrace them exactly as they are. You now begin to consciously create your outer life in a way that deeply supports the True-You.

The Three Stages of Ascension: The Octaves of Consciousness

There are typically three stages of awakening or ascension, three stages you move through as you emerge into the understanding that you are consciousness; you are pure, creative energy; and you are part of the material reality you see around you. The stages are an ascension in frequency.

Your consciousness vibrates higher and higher as you move through these stages. I learned this from a mentor of mine, Sylvie Olivier, who created Golden Heart Wisdom and greatly assisted my awakening process. She describes these stages in octaves, just like in music, where we move through the same scale over and over but in a higher frequency. It's the same world we're moving through, just seen in an entirely different way, from an entirely different vantage point. You begin to see your past experiences and the people in your life through a totally different lens as you ascend into a higher octave.

You will likely see yourself in all three stages, as we do not pop our entire being into a new octave all at once. We explore it, gain insights from it, accept more and more of it, then find ourselves bumped back into a lower octave again and again to get clarity at that level and learn. This is the way I've come to understand these stages:

First Octave of Consciousness

In the first stage or octave, you are kind of oblivious. You see yourself as physical. Everything is separate, physical stuff. Life is happening *to* you. Life is as it is, and you just have to make do with what you've got. In this level one stage, the first octave of consciousness, you try to learn the rules, go to school, study hard, be a good girl or a boy, get a good job, do the right thing, and you are going to be okay. There is a right and wrong. There are rules you have to follow, but supposedly life is going to turn out. Many of us put most of our life's energy into this. In this stage we are a victim. Life is as it is, and we have to figure out how to manage it.

If you find out you have "gotten" a disease, and it is something that is happening to you, then you have to figure out how to deal with it and what to do. You may see yourself as a victim of that disease. You may think you are not doing a good enough job or working hard enough, or are not a good enough person, or otherwise unworthy in some way. You are always scrambling to comply with the *rules* in order to survive. With these beliefs, ultimately life bumps you out of that first octave and into Stage Two, the Second Octave.

You enter Transition 1. Things get shaken up when we realize the *rules* are actually B.S. You'll hear a person in Stage One say, "I got sick," or, "My wife left me," or, "I got laid off," and they hold this as if they are an innocent bystander in the equation.

There's no awareness they are a player in the game, and things have happened as a result of who they are. Eventually, however, life shows you that the rules you thought were so hard and fast are B.S. They're Belief Systems. They are not true. No matter how hard you work, it is not going to work out. You still lost your job. You still got that disease. You have entered the Second Octave, the next level of ascension in consciousness.

Second Octave of Consciousness

You've entered the Second Octave when you realize everything you believed about everything is not true. The rules you have been taught do not work. You go through a stage of bewilderment but enter a stage of greater freedom. You realize you are part of creating what is happening to you. Something within you is part of your manifestation. You realize you are a living being who has a role in creation. Life is *responding* to you, and you interact with things in a different way.

You may learn about things like the law of attraction and how to manifest your reality. In this stage, you think: *If I could get it right, I could have things work out in my life. If I could increase my frequency, things would be okay.*

You become an active participant in life because you realize you are creative, but you are still in the identity, in the small-self. You are still in a space of fear and separation, so you try to *make it happen*, and there is attachment.

In this second octave you are still in duality, so there is right and wrong, good and bad. There's the wanted and unwanted, so you still act from attraction or aversion. You're trying to get something or avoid something. It's a tug of war. The theme of this stage is, "I must increase my frequency." You are in a higher level of awakening and freedom than Stage One, the First Octave, but you are still functioning from *fear*.

When you try with effort to create a shift and things do not work out, you think you have to do better. You might sign up for a course or go to another retreat. Self-improvement in this stage brings acceleration, but ultimately it becomes a full-time job. You may at first see some results, but ultimately you arrive at a place where you realize you are still a hamster on the wheel. You become exhausted. You realize although you may be manifesting and have some personal power, you are still working hard for it, and this is not actual freedom.

During this stage, you have more energy and awareness. You are more interactive with life and less of a victim. Things are starting to open up. You are thinking outside the box. You approach your relationships in a different way. Perhaps you are an entrepreneur, and you create a whole new way of doing something because you have taken what happened in Stage One and turned it into a gift. You use that awareness to create something beautiful, but ultimately you realize that chasing it, holding this *I am the Creator* idea is exhausting, and the temporary pseudo-freedom or pseudo-fulfillment you achieve is not the be-all and end-all of what you know in your heart is possible.

That is when you make a shift to consciously choose to ascend beyond this stage. Life is not going to do it for you. Life is not going to give you that kick in the butt like it does in Stage One. Here, you *consciously choose* to leave behind the trying and the strategies so you can ascend to the Third Octave, which is the Unknown.

In Transition 2, you have to let go. This is the leap of faith I was talking about when we move into the frequency of Love or above. It goes beyond rationality because you cannot already understand it. It does not exist in the realm of the mind and the realm of the Second Octave or in the realm of anything you have ever learned in a book or learned from someone else. This *has* to come from a space of readiness within you. This has to come from the choice to open to the unseen and the unknown power that lives inside you. Surrender must take place. This is when you move to the Third Octave.

> *I listen to the subtle nudges instead of listening to the*
> *not-so-subtle mental and emotional reactions caused*
> *by holding onto my personal preferences.*
> *This is how I practice surrender in everyday life.*
> ~ Michael Singer, *The Surrender Experiment*

Third Octave of Consciousness

In the third stage or octave, you have surrendered trying. You have surrendered attachment. You have surrendered focusing on the outer as a means to your fulfillment, and you tap into the well of life *within*. Your fulfillment is unconditional, and you create from there. Your sense of love and peace and self-acceptance are unconditional, and you choose actions from there. You create in a very different way. Instead of trying to get ahead, you allow your life to ascend in its own way and its own timing. Instead of trying to manifest what you want, you surrender and allow the expression of the *I am*, the True-Self *I*, who cannot be defined.

This is a space that cannot be learned; it can only be experienced. In this Third Octave, manifestation is instantaneous. All the experiences happening to you are for your benefit, and you receive them for your benefit. In this octave, you are in flow with life and in gratitude of everything that is happening. You are living in the True-Self, and you know it. Maybe you have experienced that. Maybe you have had a heightened experience of fluidity and freedom and joy, and something so beautiful you did not even have words for it.

You may have the thought: *I hope this lasts; I hope I stay here forever. What am I going to do to make sure I keep this going?*

Then immediately, you get bumped back into Stage Two. That attachment or control is a lower frequency. You find yourself in the Second Octave, and you feel the density of your own attachment. This becomes a *problem* because you want to keep getting back to the third stage and back to the higher consciousness. You realize you cannot *make it happen* because it already *is* happening. It already exists *here*, *now*, but you are not experiencing it because you are bumping it out. You are resisting it because you can't *manifest* your reality. You cannot *raise* your frequency. You can only surrender to be more fully in the one you are currently in. This inner surrender, however, is the *opening* that allows something higher to come into your experience.

Neutrality Bumps: How to Navigate Your Ascension

As you come through this journey, you find that point of attachment. You find yourself getting bumped out of the third stage and back into the trying-to-figure-it-out stage. I have some helpful tips for you. I have experienced this so many times and even tried to create my whole business from the Second Octave and kept falling on my face.

My work was helping people heal in amazing ways, but my business wasn't sustaining me. It wasn't thriving financially. The structure was not working out because, until I learned to live with a higher degree of surrender—letting manifestation come through me, letting life come through me, letting healing come through me—good things would happen, but they were not sustainable. Eventually, I would go back into struggle. Holding on to attachment and fear and clamping down to make things work wasn't sustainable. My life reflected where I was not truly in surrender. I had to embody more fully the I AM presence within me before I could see my life's work generate a lifestyle that truly supported me. When I finally did this, life opened up and flourished through no effort of my own.

This is one of the biggest pieces we work through in my live courses. It's a shift in consciousness. We don't see where we're still holding fear, but we do see it showing up in our lives. It's a matter of tracing that back, looking into the mirror of our deepest fear and shame and finding the courage to surrender. This is why you need to know why you are vested in your own awakening. The energies ready to release from your system will come up, and they can be very uncomfortable as they are moving out. You've got to remember what's really happening, so you choose to keep allowing the process rather than going back into contraction as a way to suppress the energy. You must let that *why*—why you are doing the work, what is your intention—be bigger than the fear. In my live course, *Embracing Health*, we transmute those fears back to pure love. We go exactly into the deepest spaces where all the lack and limitation comes from. It's there for you to reclaim your power.

Many people are ready to live from the True-Self and express it in their lives, relationships, and work. They're ready to be fully supported and sustained for who they are, instead of living as the false-self and being depleted. In my *Embracing Health* course, I show people how to get to the core of what's really creating their pain, illness, or greatest challenge and how to transmute the energies underlying it. Rather than be about a fix, this course brings people into a higher level of creatorship, power, and purpose in their lives. You are meant to live an abundant and fulfilling life, and the more you open to express the True Self, the more it always comes in.

When you sustain the I AM presence in more of your life, Life sustains you and reflects abundance in your work, money, and health. You live in sustained well-being.

How do you do this when circumstances bring you down or limitations seem to keep you stuck?

What are the keys to consistently reside in the Third Octave and live your life from there?

In this next section, I tell you about the obstacles that bump you out of Oneness Consciousness back into the Second

Octave. When I first learned about this, my mentor called that third stage *Neutrality*. This is the place where you are no longer in the good and bad, no longer in the duality. You are in the Now. You are in the All That Is. You are not in the higher or the lower. You are in total peace with All That Is. You are not in the duality of the Second Octave; it is Neutrality, Third Octave. Don't confuse this with complacency, in which things are not so good, not so bad; they're just *okay*. Oneness Consciousness or Neutrality is a state of ultimate peace and connection. It's joy and bliss.

You will know the difference between the Second Octave and the Third Octave, Neutrality, because in Stage Two you are still in duality. You are trying to get somewhere higher. You are trying to get somewhere better. You don't want to be in the lower frequency because that is *worse*. There is judgment and resistance. All of that is *duality*. It's an illusion.

In the Third Octave, you are truly in Neutrality. This is the Unity Consciousness or Oneness Consciousness, in which you are truly in the space of oneness and embracing All That Is. I used to try to live my life from there, and that just didn't work. I finally let go of trying and found the *letting go* was that higher space.

There are habits and perspectives that bump us out of Oneness and Neutrality. When we are aware of these, we have a key to catch ourselves in the act of engaging these perspectives or behaviors and can let go.

- **Neutrality Bump #1** is *attachment*. You want to stay only in the higher state. You feel a sense of lightness and immediately grasp for it because there is attachment—you do not want it to end. You are afraid it is going to go away. You have a need to control it. This is not surrender. This is not allowing. This is not letting go. It will bump you out of Oneness and back into duality. When you notice yourself wanting to *be there*, invite that feeling, invite the discord and wanting. That space of Oneness will easily come back. That is why nonattachment is important. In Stage Two, you think you can't let go, that you have to *want* it. You think you have to intend for it and hold on to it. You think you have to try or nothing else is going to manifest, but that is not true.

Let go of everything you have learned about that, and be willing to be in a state of allowing because if Neutrality, Oneness, and freedom are your natural state, you do not need to hold on to them. Let them go.

• **Neutrality Bump #2** is *judgment*. You see it as better. You want to get to a better place. You want Oneness instead. Your judgment puts you right back into duality. In this space you are going to feel the same thing. You'll have trouble getting back to the heightened space, trying to manifest the *higher* thing, trying to increase your consciousness. If you are judging it as better or superior, and you think: *ugh, I was so unconscious and stumbling around; now I know so much better*, that is superiority. Catch yourself in the act because from Oneness you are already whole. You are All That Is. You are pure love. It is all accepted. If you notice yourself in a space of judgment, you can let go of that thought or feeling and embrace where you are, as you are, how you are. The willingness to embrace *this* now moment, where you are, as you are, how you are is of Oneness. This is the Third Octave. It is a higher consciousness beyond courage. Courage is already part of your system, so you have courage enough to embrace the dense, unwanted thing, and that brings the lightness of the higher consciousness back into your moment.

- **Neutrality Bump #3** is ***trying to do it.*** You think the experience of Peace and Oneness comes *from you* and your doing. You earn it. So you ask: *What are the tools; what are the tricks? What are the strategies? How do I get there?* Thinking: *I have to do it* is another way you engage in the small-self. The small-self does not already know peace, so, of course, it thinks it has to work for it. It thinks it has to try harder or be better. Every time you are in the space of thinking: *I have to do it, I have to get it right, I have to do better,* you're identifying as the small-self. Instead remember: *Wait a minute—I already am whole, I already am what I am seeking.* Then be willing to let go of trying. Just soften your body, and you disengage the small-self.

Any time you are *trying*, it is going to bring you back into the Second Octave. Remember the Second Octave is higher than the First Octave, so the mind likes being there. It thinks *I'm getting somewhere now!*—and that's great, but when you awaken to the Truth, that's not going to be enough. Once you've known, or even heard about, what true peace and freedom are, you know too much. You won't be fooled by the Second Octave's broadcasts about how you should keep trying and pushing and eventually you'll get there. It feels too heavy.

- **Neutrality Bump #4** is *being right*. I've seen so many people, myself included, stumble on this one simply because we've invested so much into getting it right. We care deeply, so we learn, we try, we do. Maybe we've vested our lives on being a person who really gets it. When we're ready to let go of being *right*, we can let something take course that we do not already understand. Joy and love are at a higher frequency than rationality. We must surrender what we think we know in order to operate in a higher way. What if everything you've ever learned about everything is wrong? What if that learning is exactly what's keeping you from letting in everything your heart is asking for now? Are you willing to be wrong about everything you've thought and everything you've done? The ego will really not like it—and that's okay. Let's starve the ego, so we can be free.

- **Neutrality Bump #5** is *rejection*. This resistance comes from rejecting what is here—rejecting what you are experiencing right now. Whether you are feeling depressed or feeling shame and heaviness or feeling a density that is unthinkable, you think: *I do*

not even know what it is. I do not have words for it, so
it is completely rejected. You do not want to feel this
space. You are in rejection of the now, and you make
it wrong. You think: *It is wrong to feel this way. I should
not feel this way. I do not want to be here.* Rejection of
the now keeps you in jail, keeps you in duality, keeps
you in the lower frequency.

What if you could accept what you are feeling, what
you are noticing, or what you are experiencing? This
takes an immense amount of courage and willingness
because sometimes what you are feeling is *hopelessness,
helplessness, or despair,* and it makes no sense to embrace
this. It seems like it is bigger than you. You believe it
will consume you, destroy you, or get worse if you stop
fighting. There is the belief *I could never get through this.
I have to manage or medicate this or overcome this or figure
this out and escape it.*

It's very common in the current medical paradigm to see
and hear the terms *Fight Against Disease, War Against
Cancer.* This makes the circumstances bigger than us.
When you are on the ascension journey, there will be
energies you are here to embrace. Until you are willing
to embrace fear, guilt, and shame, those densities are
going to stay stuck in your system. When you find
yourself in rejection, where what you are feeling is
so unfathomable, indigestible, or impossible to let
in, have the courage to welcome everything you are
feeling, everything you are sensing, and everything you
are thinking. Even in the three deep breaths I showed

you in the Instant Elevation, you can transmute that rejection back to Love. This allows the energy to move so you can reside in a higher octave.

- **Neutrality Bump #6** is *I need to understand first.* Here you find yourself asking lots of questions: *What are you talking about? What does this mean?* You make objections and need more explanations. This comes from fear. You only embrace what you already understand. This comes from the idea that you need to control. If you do not understand, then you are not in control. To let something new in beyond what you currently understand, there has to be a level of surrender. You must surrender to the unknown, the higher space, to what you do not already understand and cannot control. When you have to first understand, you cannot go beyond that rationality. You cannot ascend into the frequency of Love or above because you need to already have the understanding.

Your brain cannot have that comprehension at the low frequency where you are. It has to open to allow the new understanding, which I promise you will come. If this form of resistance comes up for you, physically relax your body, soften your belly, and soften your shoulders. Every time you think: *I do not understand and I do not know how,* soften your physical body, take three breaths like the belly breath, surrender the moment. Let go of everything you are feeling and thinking, and you will, I promise, have higher awareness and a higher understanding than you ever could have imagined possible. But you have to surrender first and find the courage to let go.

- **Neutrality Bump #7** is *conditionality.* You do the work only to get the outcome. Making your devotion conditional keeps you stuck in duality. You are not in a state of freedom, where you already *are* that space of love, where you already *are* at peace. So you do this work to *get* peace. You surrender so you *get* freedom. You want to *get* the things you need or the feeling you want, and your attention is on the *getting*, the result. The thing is, this is very different from doing the work for the purpose of doing the work. Opening to Source is for the benefit of you living in a state of openness, living as a receiver. Surrender attachment to an outcome, and I promise when you enter the higher consciousness, all the things your heart truly desires and all the things that truly support you must manifest.

When you're surrendered, they cannot *not* come in. They cannot *not* be solved and resolved. You can let go and let yourself feel freer, feel more at ease, and feel more peace even though XYZ is happening. Sometimes, especially with EFT tapping, in which you state: *even though I am feeling this grief, even though I am in so much pain and I do not understand, I choose to embrace peace,* you have to let that choice to be at peace be *unconditional.*

- **Neutrality Bump #8** is *thinking the tools/methods are the Source.* We learn a lot that assists us on our ascension. I've personally had incredible teachers and mentors along the way who have made a massive difference in my life. I've learned and shared MindBody tools, meditations, and keys that have opened my life greatly. But as soon as I hold on to those tools as the Source, I'm back in the ego. Once we cross the river, it's time to let go of the canoe. No matter how much a tool or method may have assisted us in entering a higher consciousness, it's not the tool that is the valuable thing; it's the state we step into; it's the integration that happens, creating a pathway within us.

No matter how many awesome tools, teachings, and methods you've found to be valuable, they're only pointing you toward the truth; they are not the Truth. No matter how many amazing teachers you've learned from, the Wisdom in you is still higher. There will come a point when you've got to let go of that teacher, that method, that tool, and transcend it. The tool or teacher can only serve to open something within you. When it's time to let it go, holding on to teaching or grasping for that tool will only hold you back.

- **Neutrality Bump #9** is *having an agenda of your own.* When you hold an agenda, you have ideas about how your healing happens, when things should come into your life, or how it would go if you were in the right alignment, and here's the thing: It's all in your mind. The mind, the small-self, has all kinds of ideas about what is supposed to happen, when and how. It thinks: *Okay if I do this, then that will happen.* The Universe has its own timing about what's right for you and how and what comes to be. You can't push that. The ego certainly has its ideas: *I'm using the tools, why aren't they working?* or *I've embodied my intention over and over; something is wrong!*

This is one of the biggest impediments I've seen when people engage on this journey. When we've got our own agenda, we stay down in the Second Octave because we're still in separation and fear. True surrender means leaving behind your agenda about how, when, and what you think is supposed to happen *when you surrender*. Hold the intention, yes, but not the agenda.

• **Neutrality Bump #10** is *I do not know how.* When the small-self thinks: *I am the Creator*, you're going to struggle. This is where so many go wrong with this process. They think when we're saying "I AM a Creator" we're talking about the small-self, the identity, the one who learns and grows and gets it. That's when you become addicted to learning more self-help.

The biggest thing that had me in the pattern of illness when I did not get better, no matter what I did, was trying to know *how* to do it myself. I was trying to be a better Creator, a better manifestor. I was trying to be more powerful. I thought I needed to figure it out.

The reality is you did not create your body; you did not create your liver and your kidneys, you did not make your heart pump blood. You *cannot* do it. Once you understand that, there is a level of surrender. Sometimes people spend ten years trying harder and learning more and doing the right thing, learning from the right guru, and trying to do it better, better, better, better. Then they finally realize: *Wow, it is not possible for me to ever do this. The only thing I can do is surrender so the Intelligence can come through and do it for me.*

When you think: *I do not know how,* remember knowledge comes through you, not from you. That thought alone will invite a new level of surrender so you can let go. You do not have to do it. You are never going to figure it out. Life comes through you not from you. This thought can help neutralize the neutrality bump that keeps bumping us back into the Second Octave. When you soften your body, your brain works differently, and you realize *you* do not have to know, and something within you *does* know.

The most powerful opener when I find myself in the Second Octave is to be willing to be in the Second Octave. I became willing to love that I was sitting in shit. As soon as I was willing to be in my judgment, fear, attachment, duality, and in suffering with love, acceptance, and with presence, it always dissolved back into Oneness. It always brought me back into the space of pure love.

We've got to come back to the lightness, even if it's just the lightness that we can accept where we are. I once shared with a client, "You may find yourself lying in a pile of shit, but at least you're facing up." Is there a small way you can find the light in your densest moment?

The final thing that's been of value to me when I've found myself in the depths and doldrums of despair is to make it about something bigger. When I think I'm a singular being, the "Kim" going through something, and I want to shift it for me, that's hard. Sometimes the density that was moving through me was so much bigger, I just couldn't find the willingness to embrace it.

These were the moments when I would remember it's about Us. That I'm part of something bigger. That maybe somewhere, somehow embracing this moment with love would serve something bigger than me, would serve someone who is in even greater despair and even less capacity. I would let in the idea that we are all connected and that my compassion in that moment could be felt everywhere by everyone and make a massive difference, bigger than anything I'd imagined I could do.

These were the moments of deepest meaning. These moments opened me to another dimension of myself. These were the moments when I would find unimaginable courage and willingness and then connect with inexplicable love. I didn't know it at the time, since those moments started way back in early life, but later in life people would tell me, "You can't possibly know how much of a difference you have made in my life." And I would think: *Wow, I actually think I do.*

I am grateful we are here connecting now through this book. I'm so honored to offer you some of the tools I have found essential in navigating the journey of choosing to consciously live my life. You have taken a huge dive into consciousness and a huge inhale of a massive truth. Let yourself digest that. Let yourself sit with it. Let yourself practice it because it can only be implemented in your life and your moment and in your own navigation.

Take any of these little nuggets with you and begin practicing them. Keep what is true for you. Let go of what doesn't resonate. Try things out. Get curious. Soften your body physically. Let life lead you. Bring your attention to the space within you and surrender to what is going on outside you, even 2% more, and you will cultivate your power. I wish you the best of love and joy and expansion for every aspect and endeavor of your journey forward.

Daily Practice to Activate Your Intention:

What is your highest intention right now? What is your greatest heart's desire? Write it down here:

Example: I want to be free from pain and illness.

_____

_____

_____

_____

_____

_____

_____

_____

_____

_____

_____

_____

_____

_____

Now, *why* do you want this? Write 5 to 10 reasons why you want this manifestation, this experience, and what it will serve for you?

_____

_____

_____

_____

_____

_____

_____

_____

_____

_____

_____

_____

_____

_____

_____

_____

_____

_____

_____

_____

_____

_____

Clarify your intention. Take those 5 to 10 reasons above and feel into the energy of each one. Ask: *Who do I get to be and what do I get to experience when this intention comes about?*

See if you can feel what that feels like in your body.

Now it's a state of Being, not a hypothetical thing outside you that isn't here. Write down some notes on who you get to *be* and what you get to experience when this intention is manifested.

_____

_____

_____

_____

_____

_____

_____

_____

_____

_____

_____

_____

_____

_____

_____

_____

Center on this intention, this state of being that is the result of your intention manifesting. *Be* it now. Welcome in the sensation of it, the experience of it, the embodiment of it, and let yourself feel it physically, mentally, and emotionally.

- Where are you?

- What do you see?

- What do you smell?

- What do you hear?

- What do you feel?

- What are you doing?

Take five minutes or more a day to *be* in this place, letting in the full experience of it on every level. Feel gratitude for how awesome it is, for how real it is, for how easy it is, for the fact that it's right here, right now. Let it expand your senses, so you match the vibration of this space and consciousness.

Use the Instant Elevation Technique to cultivate this state and activate the frequency of this intention within your body every day.

Set your alarm five times a day to do the 3-Step Process, ABC. I will outline it again here. You will practice this for a few minutes in the beginning, so you generate the connections and set up this process within your system. The more you integrate this process, the more it sets up pathways so it becomes an instant process you can activate within your system anytime, just with intention. Take your time to let it integrate. It's an exponential growth curve, so at first it may seem like nothing is happening. It may seem difficult. As you install the new pathways, however, you will see more and more activation with less and less energy investment on your part. Be patient and know that you are cultivating your power.

1. A: Bring your **awareness** fully into your body. Let go of everything outside you. You can see the outer world like a chalkboard. Just erase the chalkboard, blow away the chalk dust, and call your energy back home, here, in your body. Let your energy expand out from your heart carrying your presence out as far as you like.

2. B: **Breathe** slowly and deeply with your shoulders relaxed. Let your belly balloon out with the inhales and relax back in with the exhales. You can see the breath go out beyond your body and expand out around your lower belly. Let the breath clear through your body and the area beyond your body. Take three to five slow deep breaths this way, letting your parasympathetic nervous system come back online. Yawning is a good sign.

3. C: Call in your **conscious** choice. Recall your greatest heart's desire and welcome it in, or state out loud or within yourself: *I choose to feel peace and love unconditionally,* or *I choose to live in freedom, health, and well-being, and I let go of everything that doesn't allow that.*

Make this practice your own. It will show you who you are. Use it as an access point to enter the power that is here, now for you. You are a Creator. You are free to create a life of love and to release attachment, separation, and fear. It's up to you, however, to practice your way into a new consciousness. You can create yourself as powerless and lacking. You can create yourself as full of crap and tell yourself none of this pertains to you, and you will find evidence to prove to yourself you are right. That is how powerful you are. You get to choose. It's up to you.

To consciously create the life you are truly here to live, you must entrain to the higher Truth. You can do it. It just takes practice, and the brain and nervous system will certainly begin to change. It's okay if it seems slow at first. You are on an exponential growth curve.

At first, it may seem that nothing much is changing, and the small-self may cry out: *This will take forever!* Don't believe it. Just let those thoughts be there. Before long, you will see far more powerful results with far less energy invested on your part.

The essentials you must remember in order to activate the power in this practice are:

1. You are not a physical person experiencing the physical stuff. You are the consciousness witnessing everything happening.

   You cannot be at peace as a person. You can only be at
   peace when you realize you are that which is at|
   peace already, the Self which has nothing to protect.
                                                    ~ Sunny Sharma

2. You are not separate. Divinity is always here, now, within you guiding your every moment. From wherever you are, you can access this power.

   The ability to heal deeply and with intention has always
   been ours. We must open to a new way of thinking
   and a new way of being for it is in being aware that
   all things become possible.
                                                    ~ Frank Kinslow

3. You are not powerless. Your presence and observation of anything has an impact on everyone and everything around you.

   You have a power inside of your body that affects all
   the world beyond you.
                                                    ~ Gregg Braden

When you are willing to remember and live these truths, you will live as love and access all the power of The Universe.

Conclusion

You have come through this journey into exploring and realizing the true power that lies within you. Everything is responding to your consciousness and your beliefs. Infinite possibilities exist, and reality is going to show up, reflecting what you hold within you.

Knowing that, are you ready to release resistance and be fully alive, receiving life moment to moment?

What possibilities are you ready to step into?

You have a choice. You can continue living the regular way from the outside-in, learning more, looking outside yourself, following the rules you've been taught, doing as you are told, looking to others to show you who you are and how to be, and staying on the trajectory of what has already been created. Or you can live by a new truth from the inside-out. You can recognize the creative power inside you. Everything is responding to the energy and consciousness you hold.

Living from the inside-out, you make changes by looking within, shifting within. You cultivate the energy of what you are looking for within yourself first so you are fulfilled, and that can be reflected in your reality.

You have the choice. You can take this understanding and what you have learned here and think: *This is very interesting*, march upon your merry way, and continue the regular path living from the outside-in. Or you can radically shift everything about who you are and live from the inside-out, knowing what

I have shared is true, not because science proved it, or because a doctor is showing it, or because patients all over the world are experiencing it, but because it points to a *truth within you* that you already know and that is beginning to awaken and take form.

The closure I would like you to have in completing this book is that the knowing is within you. Anything I've shared that has resonated with you is pointing you to the same truth within you, to that same knowing within you. Anything that has not fully resonated, you can let go. The truth in you is going to show you what is true for you and what is not needed. I invite you to stay in the space of knowing no matter what anyone tells you or shows you. The only things serving you are those pointing you more and more toward the *knowing* and the *strength* within you.

I invite you to make a commitment to live this truth for yourself and share it in the MindBody Community in Facebook so we can assist, encourage, and celebrate you. You can also write it on your bathroom mirror where you will see it every day and state, "I know the truth is in me and I choose to connect within for guidance and healing," or your own version of this, so you remember every day this unseen power in you.

Let this work keep speaking to you over and over. Find it within you. Focus on this daily. Let this work awaken within you daily so that you continue to live your truth more and more fully.

The final words of wisdom I will leave you with are: This truth is all in *you*, not in me, not in the book, not in teachers outside you. This book and this work are only pointing you to the truth that lies within you. That space in *you* is the source of all the wisdom that you are. Know you are the truth, and keep opening your body and mind to let that in and live it. That way, it is not conditional. You may forget what I say; you may forget what you felt while reading this; you may forget the awakening that has happened here in your body, and none of that matters.

All that matters is you keep opening now, and now, and now into that space within and let it show you everything. You are infinite. You are powerful. And, through remembering this, we, together, will create Heaven on Earth.

Next Steps

Resources, including guided audios, meditations, and videos, can be found at DrKimD.com/BYOHbonuses.

You are invited to join us in the MindBody Community group in Facebook at https://DrKimD.com/connect on Facebook to ask questions, receive assistance, and connect with others on this path.

You are also invited to join my live group program *Embracing Health* to receive live mentorship in integrating this work at DrKimD.com/health.

Let's Go Deeper

Here is what I recommend you do next:

Get FREE Gifts with this book:

Go to DrKimD.com/BYOHbonuses to receive even more support on your journey with walkthroughs of daily exercises, video demonstrations, and free meditations to enhance your healing. Plus, we'll add you to our weekly emails with MindBody TV episodes, live each week!

Go deeper on your own with the Instant Elevation Program:

Integrate the ABCs of healing. In this self-guided course, you will be guided through 21-days of establishing new circuitry in your body to integrate the ABC tool and activate powerful self-healing.

Start the home study course now at DrKimD.com/iep.

Go deeper *live* with me in the Embracing Health Program:

This is your opportunity to work with me live for a one-year integration of true health and wealth. Receive my assistance to increase your frequency and release the core root of illness, pain, and anxiety, as well as the limiting circumstances in your money, work, and relationships. Awaken your power by transmuting these energies back to pure love so you live in power and well-being.

Enrollment opens annually at DrKimD.com/health.

Connect:

Connect with like-minded souls on this expansive journey in my Facebook group The MindBody Community, on my Instagram, and through my YouTube channel at DrKimD. com/connect.

References

Byrd, R.C. 1988. "Positive Therapeutic Effects of Intercessory Prayer in a Coronary Care Unit Population." *South Med J.* Jul;81(7):826–9. doi: 10.1097/00007611-198807000-00005

Maurer, Norbet, Helmut Nissel, Monika Egerbacher, Erich Gornik, Patrick Schuller, and Hannes Traxler. 2019. "Anatomical Evidence of Acupuncture Meridians in the Human Extracellular Matris: Results From a Macroscopic and Microscopic Interdisciplinary Multicentre Study on Human Corpses." *Evidence-Based Complementary and Alternative Medicine,* vol. 2019. Article ID 6976892. 8 pages. doi.org/10.1155/2019/6976892

Rein, Glen, and Rollin McCraty. 1994. "Structural Change in Water and DNA Associated With New Physiologically Measurable States." *Journal of Scientific Exploration.* 1994; 8(3): 438–439.

About the Author

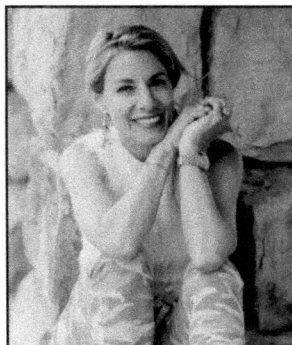

Dr. Kim D'Eramo is a physician, bestselling author of *The MindBody Toolkit*, and founder of the American Institute of MindBody Medicine. She has assisted millions in activating self-healing to resolve chronic illness.

After an awakening experience at a young age, Kim became fascinated with MindBody Medicine and spirituality, and she studied them passionately. She had the awareness she was here to be a physician and share the truth that our thoughts influence our reality, our emotions directly affect our cells, and our bodies can heal from within.

She graduated with honors from Providence College, and then attended medical school at the University of New England College of Osteopathic Medicine. It was during that time she developed a strange illness with severe joint pain, back pain, headaches, weight gain, aches, and chills all over, and she had severely low energy. When she sought help from the medical world, she was repeatedly told "nothing was wrong" and was prescribed antidepressants and other medications, until finally she was diagnosed with an autoimmune disorder.

Instead of subscribing to her doctors' perspectives and conclusions, Kim decided to investigate her own awareness about what was needed. Being highly empathic and energy sensitive, she tuned into her own inner wisdom and was able to see exactly what was limiting her health and keeping the disease in place.

Through following her own inner guidance, the illness resolved within days. Kim went on to train in Emergency Medicine at Emory University in Atlanta, where she worked at a major trauma center. This deepened her ability to trust her instincts, stay centered under immense pressure, and develop profound compassion for humanity.

Kim has now retired from Emergency Medicine and dedicated her career to sharing MindBody tools that activate the body's ability to heal itself. Her work supports her vision of a new medical system that serves those seeking healing as well as those who assist others in healing.

Kim lives with her husband and their two children in Durango, Colorado. Her work, podcast, books, and programs can be found online at DrKimD.com.

www.ingramcontent.com/pod-product-compliance
Lightning Source LLC
Chambersburg PA
CBHW062118020426
42335CB00013B/1016